Dermatologist's Handbook of Autoimmune Connective Tissue Diseases

Pooja Agarwal • Ashish Jagati
Santoshdev Rathod
Editors

Dermatologist's Handbook of Autoimmune Connective Tissue Diseases

Springer

Editors
Pooja Agarwal
Department of Dermatology
Smt. N.H.L. Municipal Medical College
Ahmedabad, Gujarat, India

Ashish Jagati
Department of Dermatology
Smt. N.H.L. Municipal Medical College
Ahmedabad, Gujarat, India

Santoshdev Rathod
Department of Dermatology
Smt. N.H.L. Municipal Medical College
Ahmedabad, Gujarat, India

ISBN 978-981-95-0523-4 ISBN 978-981-95-0524-1 (eBook)
https://doi.org/10.1007/978-981-95-0524-1

This Springer imprint is published by the registered company Springer Nature Singapore Pte Ltd.
The registered company address is: 152 Beach Road, #21-01/04 Gateway East, Singapore 189721, Singapore

Preface

Autoimmune Connective Tissue Diseases (AI-CTDs) represent a complex and evolving group of disorders that bridge multiple medical disciplines, including dermatology, rheumatology, and internal medicine. Their diverse cutaneous manifestations are often the earliest—and sometimes the only—clues to diagnosis, making dermatologists uniquely positioned to identify and manage these conditions at an early stage.

We have written this book with a vision to provide a clear, comprehensive, and clinically oriented resource on AI-CTDs. Our goal is to demystify these often daunting disorders by presenting them through the lens of cutaneous signs and patterns, while also integrating essential systemic features, diagnostic criteria, and current therapeutic strategies. We have also taken help from renowned rheumatologists for few topics, which appear to be the most confusing to a dermatologist.

Designed for postgraduate medical students as well as consultant dermatologists, this book aims to develop a deeper understanding of these diseases in both academic and clinical settings. Each chapter is structured in a way to provide concise yet thorough insights, supported by clinical photographs, tables, and illustrative diagrams for better understanding of the subject.

We hope this book serves not only as a valuable educational resource for students but also encourage deeper clinical insight and interdisciplinary collaboration. By enhancing awareness of the dermatological and systemic dimensions of autoimmune connective tissue diseases, we aim to empower the readers to recognize these conditions earlier and manage them more effectively. Ultimately, our shared goal is to improve patient outcomes through timely diagnosis, informed decision-making, and comprehensive care.

In learning, you will teach, and in teaching, you will learn. (Phil Collins)

Ahmedabad, India

Pooja Agarwal
Ashish Jagati
Santoshdev Rathod

Contents

Part I

Introduction

Introduction of Autoimmune Connective Tissue Disorders

1

Ashish Jagati and Santoshdev Rathod

Abstract

Autoimmune connective tissue diseases (AI-CTDs) comprise a heterogeneous group of disorders which have a common pathogenesis involving immune-mediated damage to the structural proteins. Dermatologists play a key role in initial recognition and management of these diseases as cutaneous manifestations are often one of the earliest clues for diagnosis. This chapter summarises the major AI-CTDs and focuses on common skin findings and targeted diagnostic approaches.

Keywords

Autoimmune · Lupus erythematosus · Systemic sclerosis · Dermatomyositis

1.1 Introduction

Autoimmune diseases are a group of disorders that involve immune responses that target 'self-antigens'. Their aetiology in most cases is unknown, but is considered to be a result of complex interaction of various genetic and environmental factors [1].

Autoimmune connective tissue diseases (AI-CTDs) are a heterogeneous group of disorders that target structural components like collagen and elastin by autoimmune mechanisms. Their prevalence in Western countries is estimated to be around 3–5% of the population. However, in Asian countries like India, the exact prevalence is not known due to paucity of demographic studies. In the last few years, the incidence has been rising in both Western and developing countries [2]. There are a

A. Jagati (✉) · S. Rathod
Department of Skin & VD, Smt SCL General Hospital, Smt NHL Municipal Medical College, Ahmedabad, Gujarat, India

P. Agarwal et al. (eds.), *Dermatologist's Handbook of Autoimmune Connective Tissue Diseases*, https://doi.org/10.1007/978-981-95-0524-1_1

wide array of diseases covered under AI-CTDs, but those having more practical relevance to the dermatologists can be broadly enlisted as [3]:

- Lupus erythematosus (LE).
- Dermatomyositis (DM) and polymyositis (PM).
- Systemic sclerosis (SS) and its variants.
- Mixed connective tissue disorder and other overlap syndrome.
- Raynaud syndrome.

1.2 Occurrence of Cutaneous Manifestations in Various AI-CTDs

Cutaneous manifestations of autoimmune connective tissue diseases are common and often paramount to diagnosis, prognosis and management. Hence, dermatologists can play a critical role in early disease recognition accelerating crucial workup and management to improve patient outcomes.

1.2.1 Lupus Erythematosus and the Skin

More than 75% LE patients present with some or the other form of cutaneous lesions during the course of their disease [4]. Around 20% of patients report cutaneous manifestations as their presenting symptom of LE [5]. Studies report that malar rash (40%), alopecia (24%) and oral ulcers (19%) are most frequent dermatologic signs [6].

1.2.2 Dermatomyositis and the Skin

Skin manifestations may precede, co-present or follow the onset of muscle involvement by months or several years. They are one of the most active and difficult features to manage [4]. Also, cutaneous manifestations of dermatomyositis tend to have a negative impact on patient's quality of life comparable to patients with psoriasis, atopic dermatitis or vitiligo [7]. Adult onset dermatomyositis, especially during the initial few years of diagnosis, was found to be linked with six fold higher risk of malignancy as compared to the general population [8, 9]. Worsening of cutaneous manifestation or recurrences are markers of underlying malignancy [10].

1.2.3 Systemic Sclerosis and the Skin

According to the literature review, cutaneous manifestations like Raynaud's phenomenon and tightening or hardening of skin are the commonest presenting symptom as compared to the respiratory (dyspnoea) or gastrointestinal (difficulty in swallowing) symptoms in scleroderma. Other common cutaneous findings are mask like facies, microstomia, pigmentary changes, narrow pinched parrot beaked nose, telangiectasias, pitted scars over finger tips, fixed flexion deformity and calcinosis cutis [11].

The spectrum of AI-CTDs is not a very fixed one and may have common cutaneous features in one or more AI-CTDs. Sometimes, AI-CTDs start as one spectrum of disease and evolve to manifest into or develop features of other AI-CTDs collectively known as 'mixed connective tissue disease'. The commonest cutaneous manifestations which give clue towards mixed connective tissue disease include Raynaud's phenomenon (78.3%), acrosclerosis (73.9%) and oedema of the hands (39.1%). Other cutaneous features including malar rash, fingertip ulceration, tightness over face, puffiness of finger and perioral paraesthesia may also be seen [12].

In various diagnostic criteria of AI-CTDs, cutaneous manifestations form one of the important criteria (major or minor) for diagnosis which signifies the importance of cutaneous examination and role of the dermatologists.

1.3 Selection of Appropriate Diagnostic Tests

In view of lesser clarity regarding the subject, it is often seen that a battery of investigations is often ordered to diagnose the disease. AI-CTDs are suspected mainly clinically, and investigations help in confirmation of the diagnosis and systemic involvement. Hence, it is preferable to do appropriate system directed practical investigations rather than using readily available anti-body panels. This would decrease the burden of laboratory investigations also. Presence of certain cutaneous features correlates with the systemic findings, and this knowledge should be used to advise the laboratory tests.

1.4 Summary

A dermatologist may find it difficult to corroborate systemic findings/complaints when they are very early or subtle making it difficult to distinguish presenting autoimmune connective tissue disease from systemic disease mimics. At a community level in a resource-limited setup, a lay person may not be aware about the rheumatologist being the specialist of these diseases, and a dermatologist would be the first point of contact in such cases based on the cutaneous features. Hence, it is important for a dermatologist to have an idea about early identification and screening of system involvement and need of prompt referral to the rheumatologist or concerned super speciality. This book contains chapters written by dermatologists and rheumatologists from specific point of view to guide management in clinical practice.

References

1. Yates DH, Miles SE. Silica and connective tissue disorders: the important role of the dermatologist. J Dermatol Skin Sci. 2022;4(2):10–9.
2. Minz RW, Kumar Y, Anand S, Singh S, Bamberi P, Verma S, Shegal S. Antinuclear antibody positive autoimmune disorders in North India: an appraisal. Rheumatol Int. 2012;32:2883–8.
3. Sterry W, Paus R, C. BWH. Dermatology. Stuttgart: Thieme; 2006.
4. Reddy BY, Hantash BM. Cutaneous connective tissue diseases: epidemiology, diagnosis, and treatment. Open Dermatol J. 2009;3(1):22–31. https://doi.org/10.2174/1874372200903010022.
5. Lee HJ, Sinha AA. Cutaneous lupus erythematous: understanding of clinical features, genetic basis, and pathobiology of disease guides therapeutic strategies. Autoimmunity. 2006;39:433–44.
6. Vitali C, Doria A, Tincani A, et al. International survey on the management of patients with SLE. I. General data on the participating centers and the results of a questionnaire regarding mucocutaneous involvement. Clin Exp Rheumatol. 1996;14(Suppl 16):S17–22.
7. Hundley JL, Carroll CL, Lang W, Snively B, Yosipovitch G, Feldman SR, et al. Cutaneous symptoms of dermatomyositis significantly impact patients' quality of life. J Am Acad Dermatol. 2006;54:217–20.
8. Olazagasti JM, Baez PJ, Wetter DA, Ernste FC. Cancer risk in dermatomyositis: a meta-analysis of cohort studies. Am J Clin Dermatol. 2015;16(2):89–98.
9. Buchbinder R, Forbes A, Hall S, Dennett X, Giles G. Incidence of malignant disease in biopsy-proven inflammatory myopathy: a population-based cohort study. Ann Intern Med. 2001;134(12):1087–95.
10. Hu T, Vinik O. Dermatomyositis and malignancy. Can Fam Physician. 2019;65(6):409–11.
11. Dave J, Mahajan S, Khadilkar P, et al. Cutaneous features, autoantibody profile, and Nailfold Capillaroscopy of systemic sclerosis: a study of 60 cases. J Assoc Physicians India. 2022;70(11):24–3.
12. Sen S, Sinhamahapatra P, Choudhury S, Gangopadhyay A, Bala S, Sircar G, Chatterjee G, Ghosh A. Cutaneous manifestations of mixed connective tissue disease: study from a tertiary care hospital in eastern India. Indian J Dermatol. 2014;59(1):35.

Dermoscopy in Autoimmune Connective Tissue Diseases (AI-CTD)

2

Hita Mehta and Manal Dave

Abstract

The potential of dermoscopy for assessing skin lesions associated with AI- CTDs remains unexplored. Within this chapter, the dermoscopic aspects of connective tissue disorders are elaborated upon and categorized into sections covering inflammoscopy, trichoscopy, and nailfold capillaroscopy. Some indicators are useful not only for diagnosis but also for monitoring the therapeutic response such as reduction in follicular keratotic plugs in chronic cutaneous lupus erythematosus after treatment.

Trichoscopic abnormalities may be present in connective tissue disease patients even in the absence of visible clinical signs, where trichoscopy helps in early diagnosis. Nailfold capillaroscopy is useful in evaluating the severity and prognosis of AI- CTDs especially systemic sclerosis. This chapter contributes to the existing knowledge and anticipates that further studies will yield more valuable insights in the dermoscopy of cutaneous lesions of connective tissue disease.

Keywords

Dermoscopy · Connective tissue disease · Inflammoscopy · Trichoscopy · Nailfold capillaroscopy

H. Mehta (✉)
Department of Dermatology, Venereology, and Leprosy, Government Medical College, Bhavnagar, Gujarat, India

M. Dave (✉)
Senior Resident, Department of Dermatology, Venereology, Leprosy Government Medical College, Bhavnagar, Gujarat, India

P. Agarwal et al. (eds.), *Dermatologist's Handbook of Autoimmune Connective Tissue Diseases*, https://doi.org/10.1007/978-981-95-0524-1_2

Abbreviations

NFC	Nail fold capillaroscopy
ACLE	Acute cutaneous lupus erythematosus
SCLE	Subacute cutaneous lupus erythematosus
CCLE	Chronic cutaneous lupus erythematosus
LET	Lupus erythematosus tumidus
DM	Dermatomyositis
SS	Systemic sclerosis
SLE	Systemic lupus erythematosus
CTD	Connective tissue disease

2.1 Introduction

Dermoscopy is a simple, rapid, reliable, and non-invasive diagnostic tool that enables the visualization of morphological characteristics that are not visible to the naked eye, bridging the gap between macroscopic clinical dermatology and microscopic dermatopathology [1]. Auto-immune connective tissue diseases (AI-CTDs) have varied clinical presentations affecting the skin, hair, and nail folds. Dermoscopy plays a crucial role in the diagnosis of AI-CTDs. Nailfold capillaroscopy (NFC) has been widely described for systemic sclerosis (SS) and is a part of the ACR EULAR criteria for the diagnosis of the disease, and NFC is also useful in evaluating the severity and prognosis of SS.

While dermatomyositis may show a similar pattern to SS, such specific findings are not found in other AI-CTDs. Furthermore, there is limited literature available that describes the dermoscopy of skin and hair changes in AI-CTDs.

Dermoscopic findings aid in the diagnosis and differentiation of disorders that imitate connective tissue disorders. This chapter describes the dermoscopy of connective tissue disorders under the headings of inflammoscopy, trichoscopy, and nailfold capillaroscopy.

2.2 Inflammoscopy

- Inflammoscopy refers to the dermoscopy of the inflammatory conditions.
- The dermoscopy of the inflammatory conditions can be described under the following parameters: vessels, scales, background, follicular findings, pigmentary changes, and other specific clues. In patients with dark skin type, the presentation of vascular structures, background colour, and pigmentary changes varies compared to those with lighter skin.

2.2.1 Lupus Erythematosus

- According to the Duesseldorf classification, there are four clinical types of cutaneous LE, acute cutaneous LE (ACLE), subacute cutaneous LE (SCLE), chronic

ACLE	SCLE	CCLE	LET
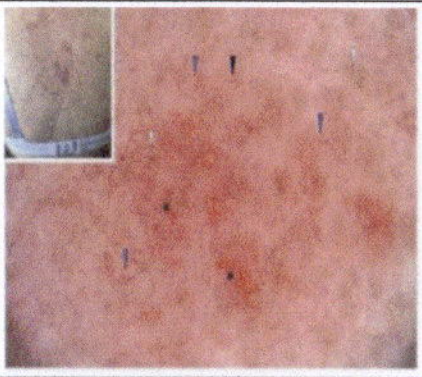	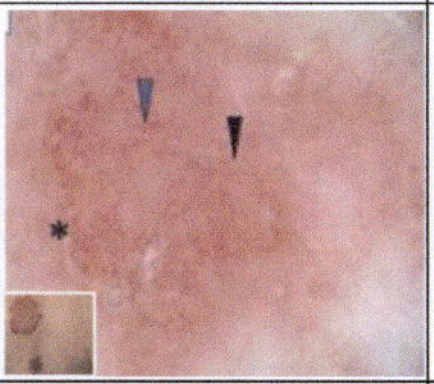	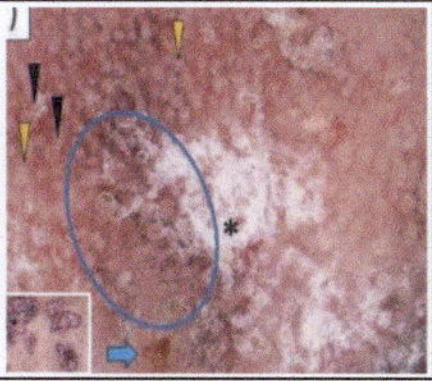	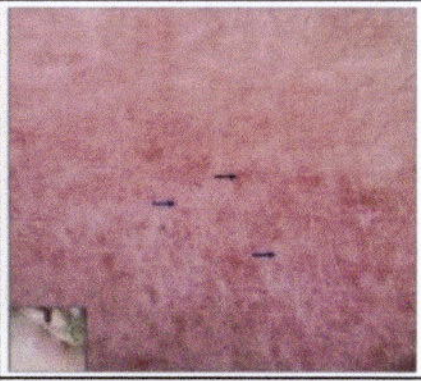
Linear (black arrow head) and linear branched vessels (blue arrowhead), follicular plugs (white arrowhead) and red structureless (haemorrhagic) areas (black asterisk). Image reference(3)	Discrete peripheral scaling (black asterisk) and abundance of linear (blue arrowhead) and linear branched (black arrowhead) vessels on pink background Image reference(3)	White scaling (black asterisk), follicular plugs (black arrowhead), white perifollicular halo (yellow arrowhead), gray–brown dots (blue circle) and erosion (blue arrow). Image reference(3)	Pinkish red background with white structureless area (blue arrow) and irregular vessels (black arrow) which are more marked in LET

Fig. 2.1 Cutaneous lupus erythematosus

Early lesion of malar rash	Late lesion of malar rash	Normal face
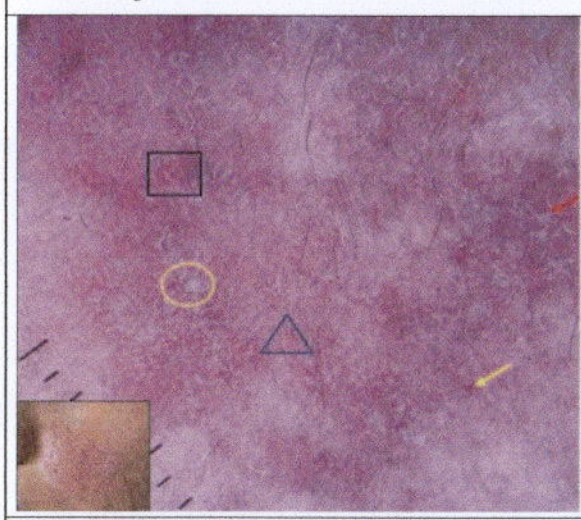	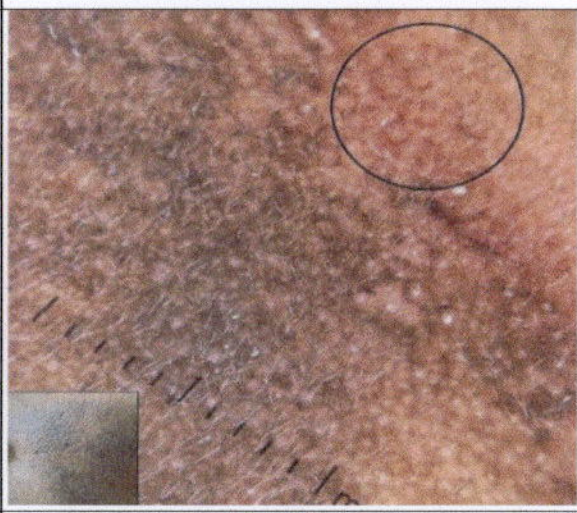	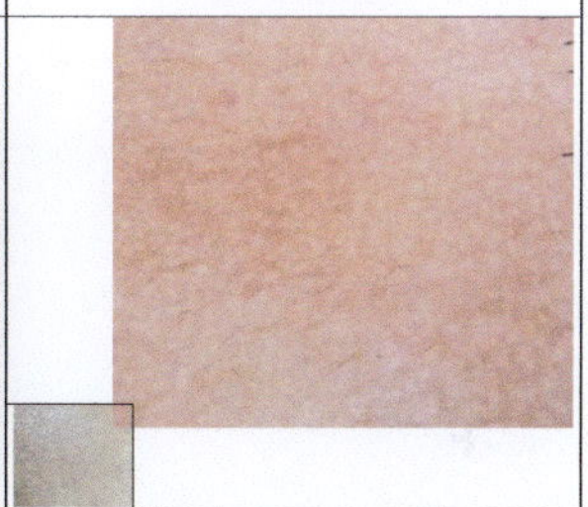
Pinkish background with red lines (black square), red dots (yellow arrow), keratotic plug (yellow circle), brown dots (blue triangle) and scale(red arrow).	Brownish background with the vascular network at the periphery (black circle).	Pseudo reticular network

Fig. 2.2 Dermoscopy of malar rash and normal face

cutaneous LE (CCLE), and intermittent cutaneous LE (lupus erythematosus tumidus (LET)). Their dermoscopic features are shown in Fig. 2.1 [2, 3].

2.2.1.1 Acute Cutaneous Lupus Erythematosus: Fig. 2.2

- Generalized: White scaling, pinkish-white to reddish-white background, brown dots and globules, keratotic plugs, and linear or linear branched vessels with a few dotted vessels.
- Localised (malar rash): Early lesion shows erythematous background with telangiectasia, while late shows vascular network with pigmentary changes. The differential diagnosis of malar rash is depicted in Fig. 2.3 [4].

Melasma	Seborrheic Dermatitis	Rosacea	CCLE
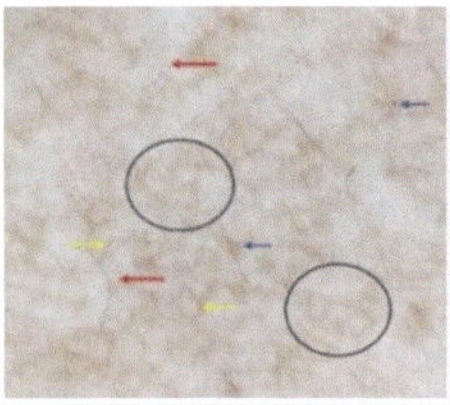	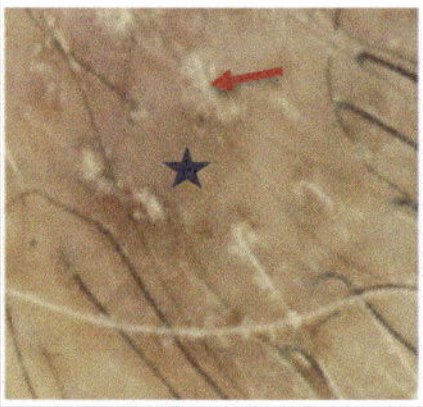	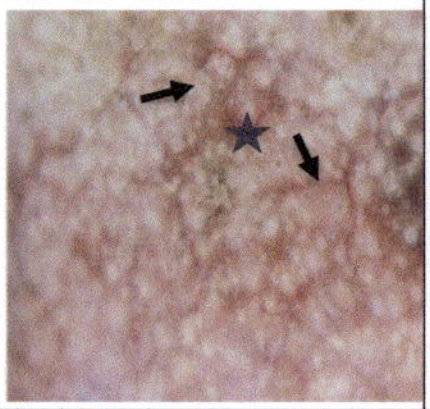	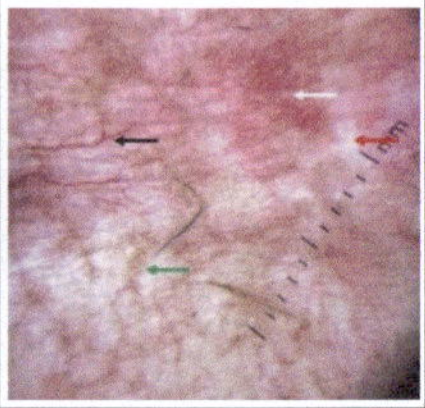
Pseudo reticular network (black circles) with perifollicular sparing (red arrow), brown dots and globules (blue arrow), arcuate structure (yellow arrow)	Pinkish brown background (blue star), and yellow scales (red arrow)	Red coloured background (blue star) arborizing vessel with as-reticular vascular like pattern (black arrow)	Pinkish red background (white arrow) with irregular branching vessels (black arrow), white structureless area (red arrow) and pigmentary network (green arrow)

Fig. 2.3 Differential diagnosis of malar rashes

SCLE	Lichen Planus
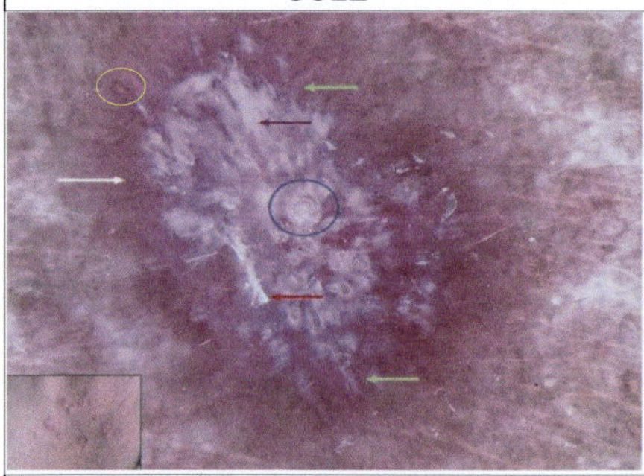	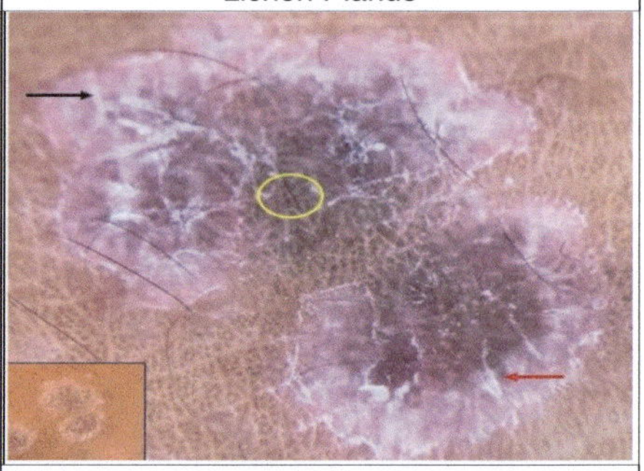
Pinkish background with discrete white scales (red arrow), follicular hyperkeratosis (blue circle), white structureless area (purple arrow) and irregular dotted vessels (white arrow) and hairpin vessel (yellow circle)	Violaceous to brownish background with brown globules (yellow circle), scales (red arrow), Wickham's striae (black arrow) and no vascular structure

Fig. 2.4 Differential diagnosis of SCLE with clinically mimicking lichen planus

- Dermoscopic features are more pronounced in early and well-developed lesions of ACLE.

2.2.1.2 Subacute Cutaneous Lupus Erythematosus: Fig. 2.4

- Whitish scaling and a vascular pattern with at least two types of vessels (linear, linear- irregular, branching, and sparsely scattered dotted vessels) on pinkish-red background.

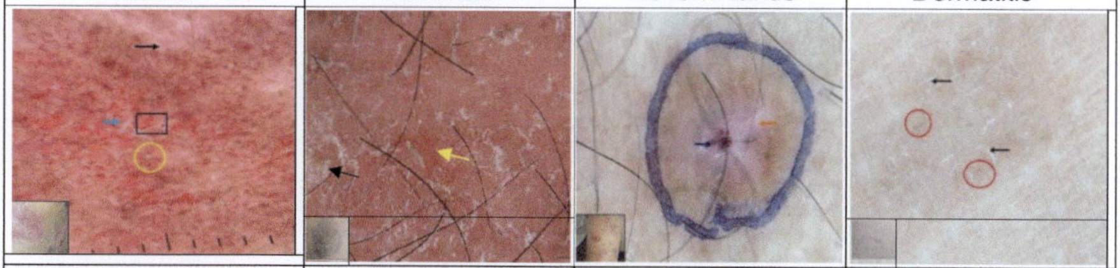

CCLE	Psoriasis	Lichen Planus	Dermatitis
White structureless area (black arrow), irregular vessels (black square), white streak (light blue arrow) and follicular hyperkeratosis (yellow circle)	Pinkish background with regular dotted vessels (yellow arrow) and white scales (black arrow)	Wickham's striae (orange arrow) and irregular red dots (dark blue arrow)	Discrete scales (black arrow) and irregular brown dots (red circle)

Fig. 2.5 Differential diagnosis of CCLE

- It is differentiated from chronic cutaneous lupus erythematosus (CCLE) by the absence of keratotic plugs, dilated follicles, and perifollicular whitish halos and the monomorphic vascular pattern.

2.2.1.3 Chronic Cutaneous Lupus Erythematosus: Fig. 2.5

- Early lesions: Follicular keratotic plugs, serving as an indicator of disease activity and therapy monitoring in patients with CCLE [5].
- Older lesions: White structureless areas and honeycomb pigmentary network.
- Vascular changes can be seen in both active and older lesions which are hallmark of CCLE.
- Follicular keratotic plug which corresponds clinically to adherent scales, follicular whitish halo to depigmentation, short linear vessels to telangiectasia, structureless white area to scarring/atrophy, and pigmentation to hyperpigmentation.
- Disseminated CCLE also shows dermoscopic findings similar to the localized lesions.
- The common differential diagnosis for CCLE includes psoriasis, lichen planus, and dermatitis, as shown in Fig. 2.5.

2.2.1.4 Mucosal CCLE: Fig. 2.6

- The hallmark dermoscopic features of mucosal CCLE include scaling, prominent white structureless area, while erosions and irregular vessels are more prominent in other conditions.

Lip CCLE	Lip Lichen planus	Lip Pemphigus Vulgaris
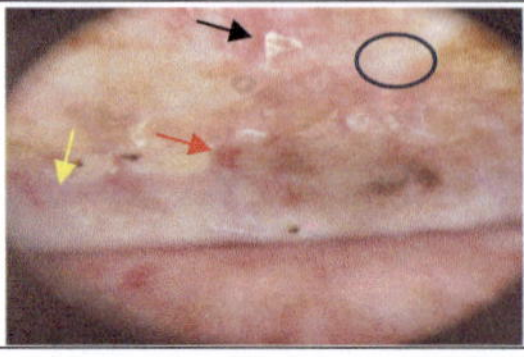	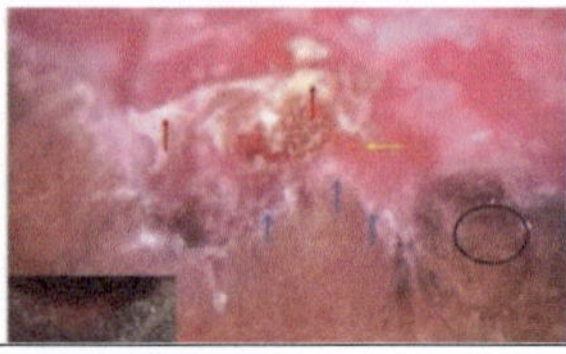	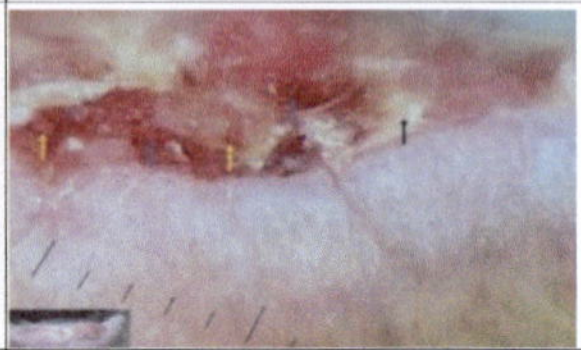
Scaling (black arrow), white structureless area (blue circle), erosion (red arrow) irregular vessel (yellow arrow)	Linear Wickham's striae(blue arrow), vessels(yellow arrow), scales(red arrow), brown pigmentation(black circle)	Ulcer and erosion (blue arrow), vessels(yellow arrow) and scales(black arrow)

Fig. 2.6 Mucosal lesions of CCLE with differential diagnosis

Gottron's Papule(6)	V neck sign	Heliotrope rash	Calcinosis Cutis
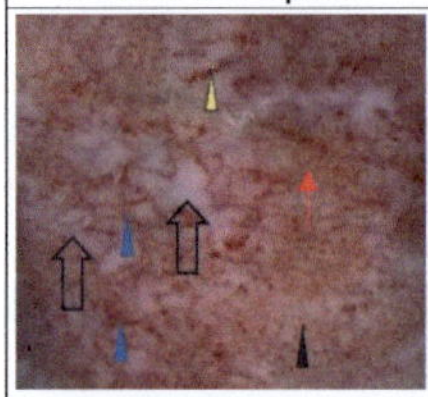	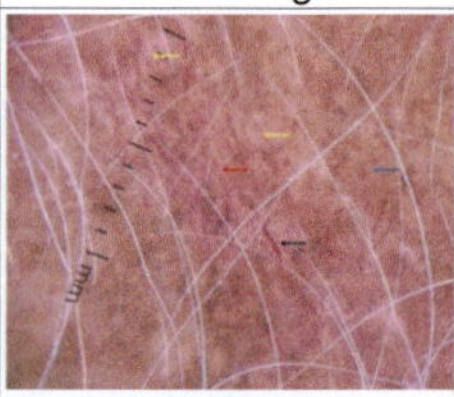	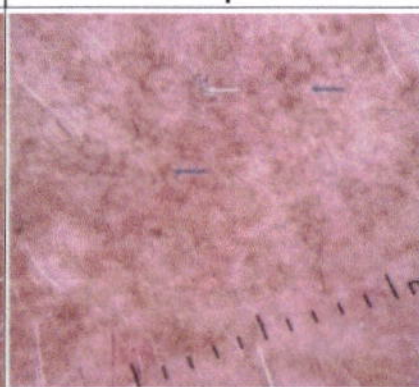	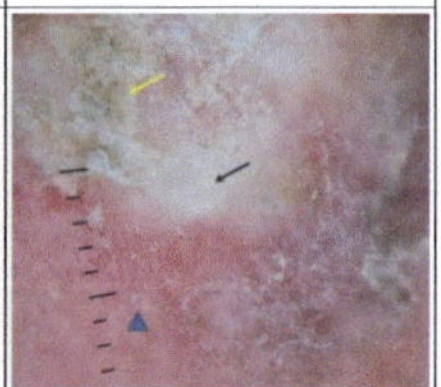
Dotted and linear vessels with branches (black and blue arrowhead), and linear curved vessels (yellow arrowhead) white structureless areas (black arrow) and scales (red arrow) Image reference(6)	Pinkish background (red arrow), white structureless area (yellow arrow), irregular vessels (black arrow) and broken pigmentary network (blue arrow)	Brownish pseudo reticular network (blue arrow), scales (white arrow) on pinkish background	White structureless area(black arrow), yellowish scales (yellow arrow) on pinkish background(blue triangle)

Fig. 2.7 Dermoscopy of dermatomyositis lesions [6]

2.2.2 Dermatomyositis: Fig. 2.7

2.2.3 Systemic Sclerosis

The matted pattern of telangiectasia is frequently detected in patients with anticentromere Ab, while the stellate pattern is seen in patients with anti-topoisomerase I Ab [7] (Fig. 2.8).

- Dermoscopy of salt and pepper pigmentation on limbs and neck: The dermoscopy can be a useful tool in differentiating salt and pepper pigmentation in systemic sclerosis from other similar looking conditions such as vitiligo and lichen sclerosus et atrophicus [8] as shown in Fig. 2.9.

Face	Hands–Matted	Hands -Stellate	Digital ulcer
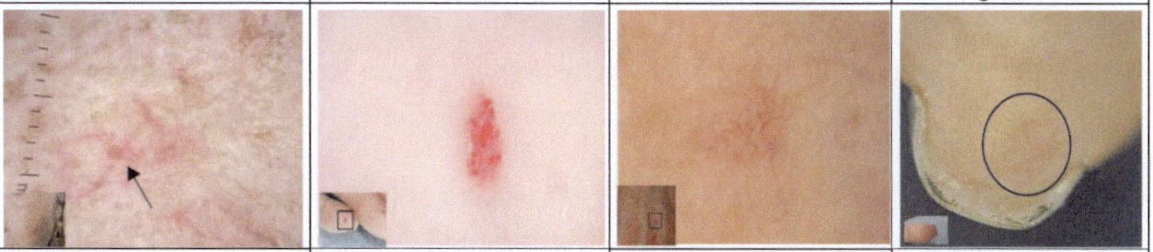			
Arborizing telangiectasia (black arrow)	Matted telangiectasia (Well-circumscribed dense telangiectasis) Image reference(7)	Stellate telangiectasia (Poorly-marginated linear telangiectasis) Image reference(7)	Homogenous brown area suggestive of pitted scar (black circle)

Fig. 2.8 Dermoscopy of different lesions in systemic sclerosis

Salt and Pepper pigmentation	Vitiligo	Lichen Sclerosuset Atrophicans	Morphea
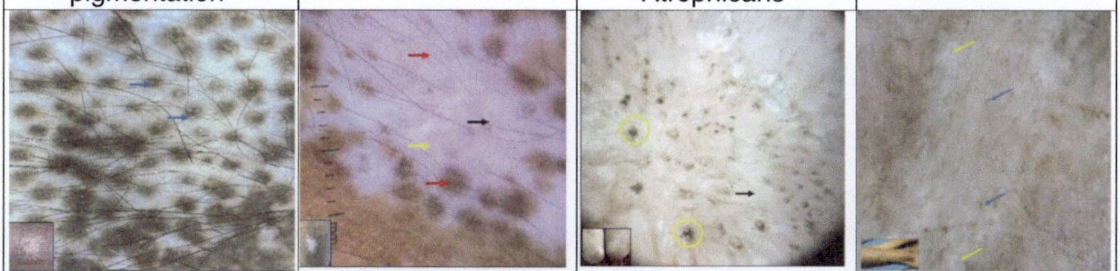			
Perifollicular dark pigmentation (blue arrow). Also, there is appearance of pepper sprinkled on bed of salt	Absent pigmentary network (yellow arrow), perifollicular pigmentation and depigmentation (red arrow), leukotrichia (black arrow)	Chrysalis like structure (black arrow) and comedo like opening (yellow circle)	White fibrotic beams (yellow arrow) & brown dots (blue arrow)

Fig. 2.9 Dermoscopy of salt and pepper pigmentation with differential diagnosis

Salt and pepper appearance of the skin could be the early and alone feature of the SS without sclerosis of the skin [9]. In such scenario it can be easily picked up on dermoscopy.

2.3 Trichoscopy

- Trichoscopy is the dermoscopic assessment of hair and scalp changes.
- Trichoscopic abnormalities may be present in CTD patients even in the absence of visible signs; hence, knowledge of their distinguishing characteristics may be of considerable benefit when there is a diagnostic challenge [10].

2.3.1 Systemic Lupus Erythematosus

- Hair changes in lupus can be lupus hair or cicatricial alopecia in CCLE of scalp.
- Trichoscopic features of scarring lesions of CCLE and its differential are shown in Fig. 2.10.
- Dermoscopy helps identify the area of disease activity of CCLE scalp lesions and thus also helps in deciding the site for biopsy.

2.3.2 Dermatomyositis: Fig. 2.11

- Pigmentation: Perifollicular red brown pigmentations and blue grey speckled pigmentation.
- Vascular changes are more commonly observed in the perifollicular region [10].
- Pinkish background.

2.3.3 Systemic Sclerosis: Fig. 2.11

- White patches between normal follicular units due to fibrosis and microcirculation insufficiency [10].
- Perifollicular hypopigmentation.
- Background vessels (Fig. 2.12).

Scalp CCLE	Lichen plano pilaris	Pseudopelade of brocq
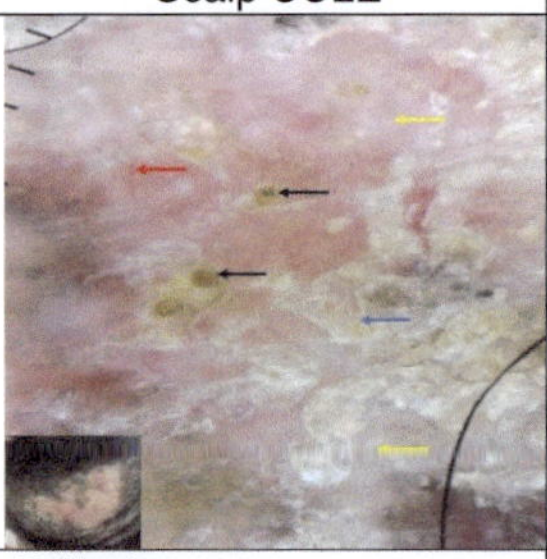	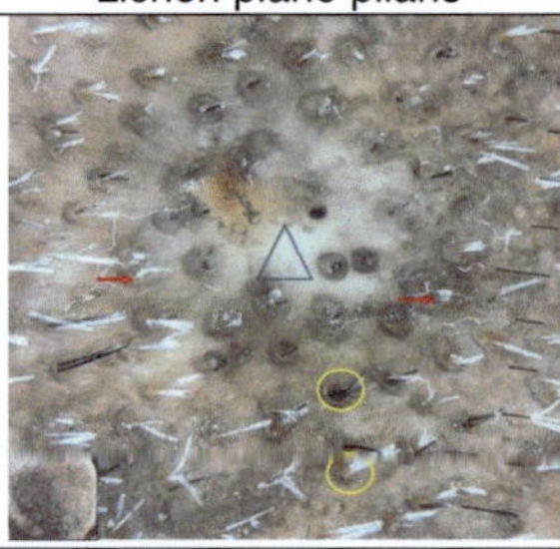	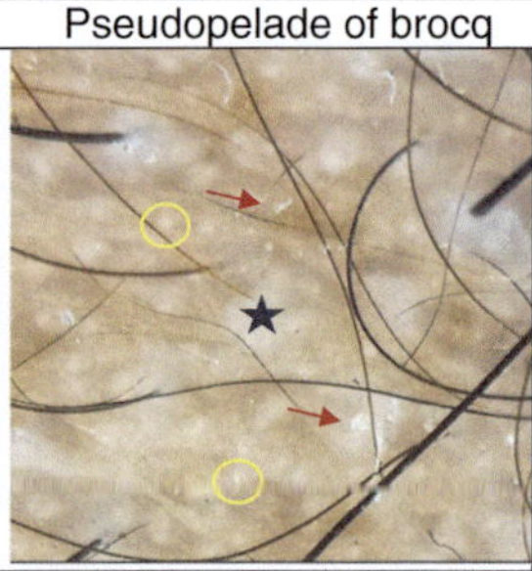
Follicular hyperkeratosis (black arrow)	Peripilar scales (red arrow)	Empty follicular ostium (yellow circle)
Tortuous vessels are markedly present (red arrow)	Vessels not markedly present	Vessels not seen
Dark brown to blue-grey pigment pattern in the interfollicular area[4].	Pigmentation is around the follicles[4].	Interfollicular Patchy pigmentation and white structureless areas (blue star)
Scales (blue arrow) and white structureless area (yellow arrow)	Tuft of 2-3 hairs (yellow circle),loss of follicular opening (blue triangle)	Occasional white scales (red arrow)

Fig. 2.10 Trichoscopy of scalp CCLE and its differential diagnosis

SLE	DM	SS
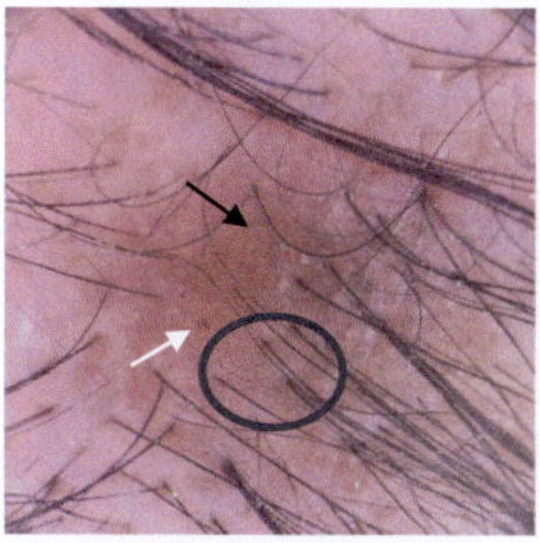	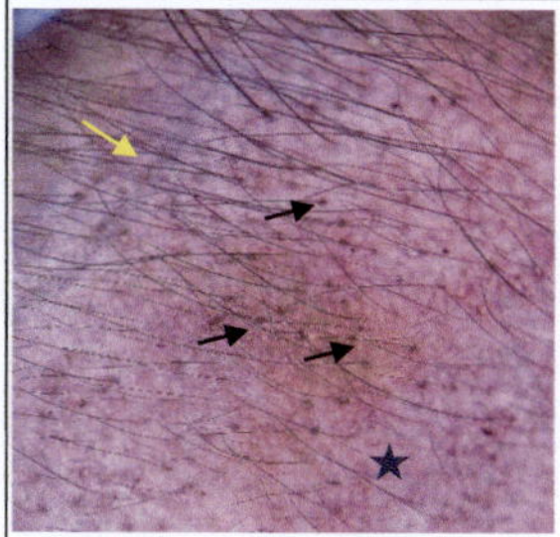	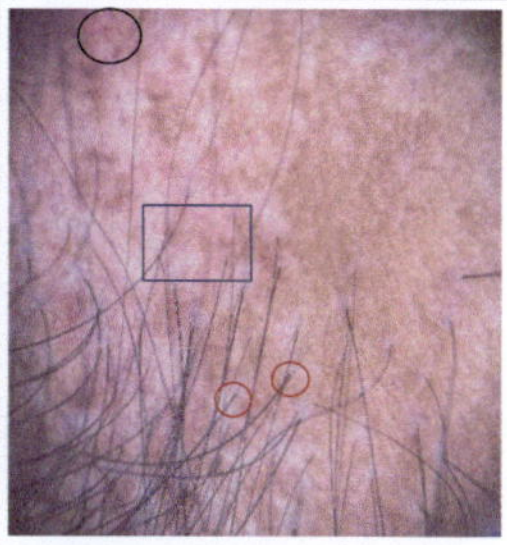
Brown pigmentation (black arrow), empty follicle (white arrow) hair shaft diameter variability.	Pinkish Background (blue star) Perifollicular red-brown speckled pigmentation (black arrow) vessels at periphery (yellow arrow)	White-brown patches (blue square) vessel (blue circle) perifollicular hypopigmentation (red circle)

Fig. 2.11 Trichoscopic features of non-scarring lesions of SLE, DM, and SS

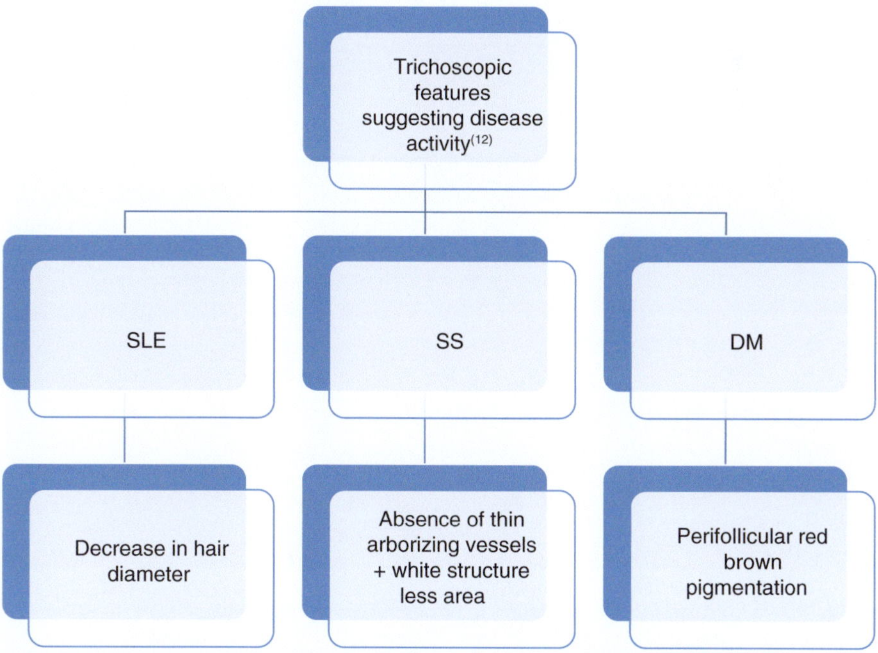

Fig. 2.12 Trichoscopic features suggesting disease activity in SLE, SS, and DM

2.4 Nailfold Capillaroscopy

The capillary alterations observed through the dermoscope not only aid in diagnosis but also assist in evaluating disease severity, therapeutic response, and prognosis. We should look for the features mentioned in Fig. 2.13 in the nailfold while suspecting connective tissue disease. Nailfold capillaroscopy (NFC) can be performed using a handheld dermoscope or a USB dermoscope, but the latter is more efficient in observing capillaries, which are essential for the diagnosis of CTD.

NFC patterns are described in the following categories [11] as shown in Fig. 2.14.

1. Non-scleroderma pattern: (a) normal, (b) nonspecific abnormalities.
2. Sclerodermoid pattern: (a) early, (b) active, (c) late.

2.4.1 Systemic Lupus Erythematosus

1. SLE: tortuous capillaries, elongated capillaries, and prominent subpapillary plexus.
2. Higher SLEDAI (SLE disease activity index) scores are associated with the presence of enlarged capillaries, which is indicative of disease activity [11].
3. Chilblain lupus: tortuous capillaries, enlarged capillaries, and/or microhaemorrhages over a reddish/purple background [12].

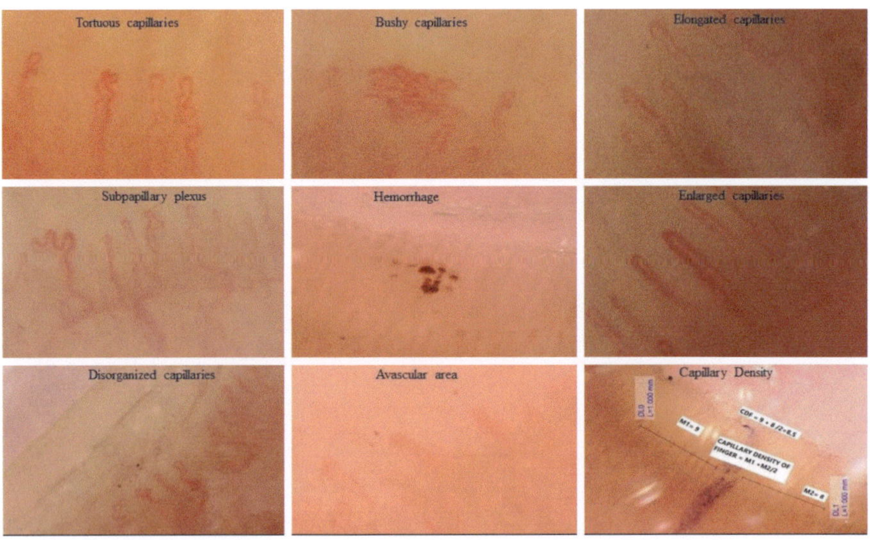

Fig. 2.13 Nailfold capillaroscopy features to be observed while suspecting CTD

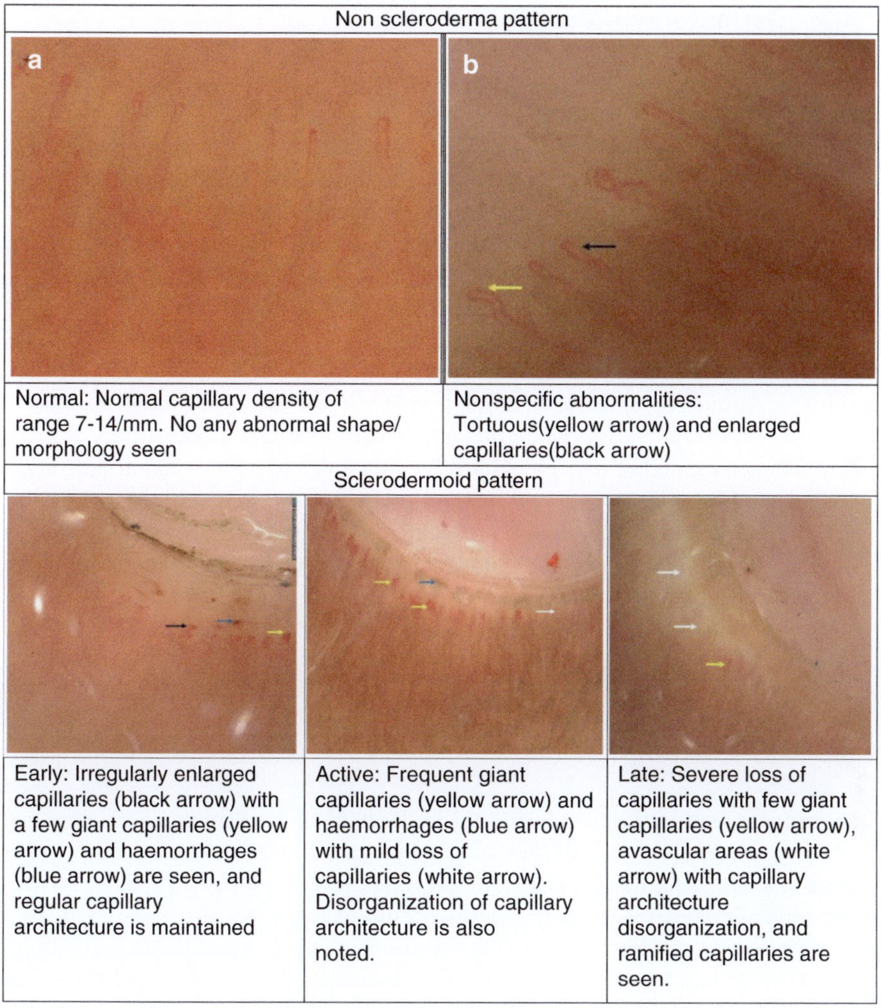

Fig. 2.14 NFC of non-scleroderma and sclerodermoid pattern

2.4.2 Systemic Sclerosis

- The NFC pattern of SS can be divided into three categories as shown in Fig. 2.14.
- Capillary loss is associated with disease severity and vascular manifestations such as digital ulcers, calcinosis, and pulmonary arterial hypertension [13].
- Patients with active and late patterns should be screened for interstitial lung disease; thus NFC aids in monitoring the organ involvement in SS [14].

2.4.3 Dermatomyositis

- DM is considered a scleroderma spectrum condition. It shares nailfold capillaroscopic characteristics similar to SS.
- However, the presence of a bushy capillary is an important NFC finding that indicates a higher likelihood of DM compared to SS [11].
- Capillary morphology findings such as tortuosity, dilated, meandering, bushy capillaries, etc. can be found in isolated fingers in healthy individuals [15], but their presence in more than one finger may raise a suspicion of diseases like CTDs.
- The absence of vascular areas is mild in SLE, mild to moderate in DM, and moderate to severe in SS [11].
- NFC can serve as both a diagnostic tool and a prognostic indicator for CTDs.
- From a dermoscopy and histopathology perspective, white scales correspond to hyperkeratosis, while vascular structures to vasodilatation of the vessels, follicular dots correspond to perifollicular inflammation, and white structureless areas correspond to oedema or fibrosis and, in some cases, mucin deposition.
- The keratotic plug corresponds to follicular hyperkeratosis, orange yellow areas to hemosiderin deposition, and pigmentary structures to melanin incontinence or basal layer pigmentation [16].
- Dermoscopy allows for improved visualization of vessels, colour variations, and scales that are hard to discern with the naked eye.

2.5 Conclusion

Dermoscopic features are a valuable aid in the clinical assessment of autoimmune connective tissue diseases (AICTDs). They help in differentiating clinically similar conditions, assessing disease activity, and monitoring treatment response. In systemic lupus erythematosus (SLE), dermoscopy distinguishes the malar rash from acne rosacea and melasma by showing the absence of polygonal vessels and a pigment network, and by presence of follicular keratotic plugs, scales, and vessels as dots and lines. In nailfold capillaroscopy (NFC), capillary loss correlates with disease severity and vascular manifestations. Patients with active and late NFC patterns should be screened for interstitial lung disease. Thus, NFC plays an important role in monitoring systemic involvement in systemic sclerosis (SS) (Fig. 2.15). In dermatomyositis (DM), dermoscopy reveals prominent vascular changes, which reflect the underlying perivascular inflammatory infiltrates.

SLE	DM	SS
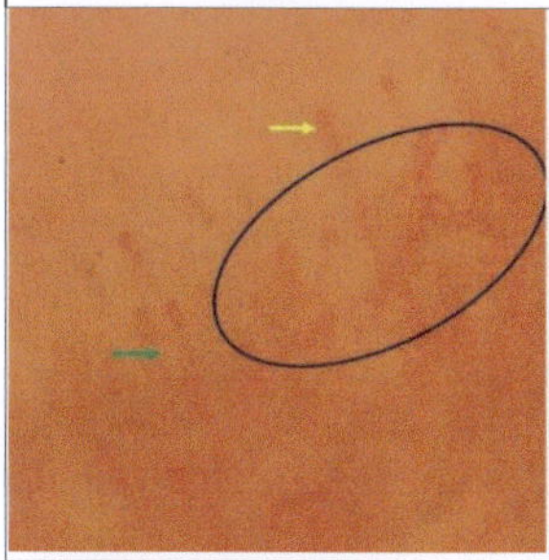	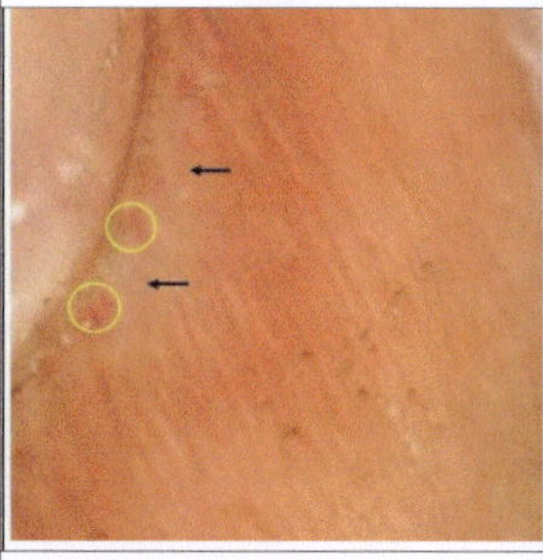	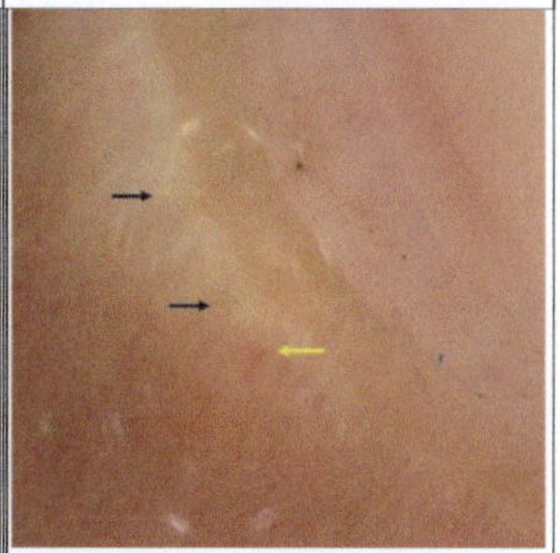
Elongated capillaries (yellow arrow), tortuous capillaries (green arrow) and prominent subpapillary plexus (black circle)	Avascular area (black arrow) and bushy capillaries (yellow circle)	Avascular area (black arrow) and disorganized capillaries (yellow arrow)

Fig. 2.15 NFC of SLE, DM, and SS

References

1. Nayak SS, Mehta HH, Gajjar PC, Nimbark VN. Dermoscopy of general dermatological conditions in Indian population: A descriptive study. Clin Dermatol Rev. 2017;1(2):41.
2. Kuhn A, Landmann A. The classification and diagnosis of cutaneous lupus erythematosus. J Autoimmun. 2014;48-49:14–9.
3. Żychowska M, Reich A. Dermoscopic Features of Acute, Subacute, Chronic and Intermittent Subtypes of Cutaneous Lupus Erythematosus in Caucasians. J Clin Med. 2022;11(14):4088. PMID:35887849 PMCID:PMC9321208.
4. Kang IH, Seo JK, Shin MK. Useful dermoscopic findings for differentiating rosacea from seborrheic dermatitis. Indian J Dermatol. 2020;65(4):316–8. https://doi.org/10.4103/ijd.IJD_44_19. PMID: 32831379; PMCID: PMC7423217.
5. Al-Refu K. The role of dermoscopy in assessment of the activity and scarring response in discoid lupus erythematosus. Open Dermatol J. 2018;12(1)
6. Żychowska M, Reich A. Dermoscopy and Trichoscopy in Dermatomyositis-A Cross-Sectional Study. J Clin Med. 2022;11(2):375. https://doi.org/10.3390/jcm11020375. PMID: 35054069; PMCID: PMC8778875.
7. Hasegawa M. Use of dermoscopy in the evaluation of connective tissue diseases. Dermatol Clin Res. 2015;1(3):41–8.
8. Bains A, Rajagopal SV, Lahoria U. Dermoscopy of salt and pepper pigmentation. Indian Dermatol Online J. 2022;13(4):548–50.
9. Singh A, Ambujam S, Varghese A, Vishranth SP, Sadanandan N. Salt-and-pepper appearance: a cutaneous clue for the diagnosis of systemic sclerosis. Indian J Dermatol. 2012;57(5):412.
10. Chanprapaph K, Limtong P, Ngamjanyaporn P, Suchonwanit P. Trichoscopic signs in dermatomyositis, systemic lupus erythematosus, and systemic sclerosis: A comparative study of 150 patients. Dermatology. 2022;238(4):677–87.
11. Chanprapaph K, Fakprapai W, Limtong P, Suchonwanit P. Nailfold capillaroscopy with USB digital microscopy in connective tissue diseases: A comparative study of 245 patients and healthy controls. Front Med. 2021;8:683900.

12. Lambertini M, et al. Chilblain lupus with nail involvement: A case report and a brief overview. Skin Appendage Disord. 2018;5(1):42–5. https://doi.org/10.1159/000488543.
13. Repa A, Avgoustidis N, Kougkas N, Bertsias G, Zafiriou M, Sidiropoulos P. Nailfold videocapillaroscopy as a candidate biomarker for organ involvement and prognosis in patients with systemic sclerosis. Mediterr J Rheumatol. 2019;30(1):48–50.
14. Smith V, Distler O, Du Four T, Cutolo M. Is there a role for nailfold videocapillaroscopy in interstitial lung disease? Rheumatology. 2022;61(6):2217–20.
15. Gorasiya AR, et al. Nailfold Capillaroscopy of healthy individuals – An observational study. Indian Dermatol Online J. 2022;13(5):600–5. https://doi.org/10.4103/idoj.idoj_80_22.
16. Ankad BS, et al. Implications of dermoscopy and histopathological correlation in discoid lupus erythematosus in skin of color. Indian J Dermatol. 2022;67(1):5–11. https://doi.org/10.4103/ijd.ijd_591_21.

Autoantibodies: Antinuclear Antibodies (ANAs) and Extractable Nuclear Antigen (ENA) 3

Rutviz Mistry

Abstract

Autoantibodies are the main culprit behind causing various autoimmune connective tissue diseases. Their detection and interpretation form a cornerstone in diagnosis of these diseases. Usually they are not associated with predicting the course of disease, but a few of them are associated with characteristic cutaneous or systemic features, and hence their knowledge is paramount.

Keywords

Antinuclear antibodies · Autoantibodies · Nuclear pattern

3.1 Introduction

Antinuclear antibodies (ANAs) are a group of autoantibodies that target varied antigens among the components of the cell nucleus [1].

- ANAs are commonly detected in the blood of individuals with autoimmune diseases, including systemic lupus erythematosus (SLE), Sjögren's syndrome (SS), Systemic sclerosis (SSc), Dermatomyositis (DM), and Mixed Connective Tissue Disease (MCTD).
- For decades, ANA testing has been an important tool in the diagnosis of these diseases, as well as other conditions such as Autoimmune Hepatitis and Drug-

R. Mistry (✉)
Rheumatology Clinic, Ahmedabad, Gujarat, India

Department of Rheumatology, GMERS Sola, Ahmedabad, Gujarat, India

Consultant Rheumatologist, KD Hospital, Ahmedabad, Gujarat, India

P. Agarwal et al. (eds.), *Dermatologist's Handbook of Autoimmune Connective Tissue Diseases*, https://doi.org/10.1007/978-981-95-0524-1_3

induced lupus. It has become a routine assay in the diagnosis of autoimmune diseases.
- Despite the clinical utility of ANA testing, there is a great deal of complexity surrounding the interpretation of ANA results. There are multiple methods for ANA testing, and the interpretation of ANA patterns can be challenging due to their varied association with specific autoimmune diseases.
- A positive ANA test *does not* necessarily indicate the presence of an autoimmune disease, as ANAs can also be found in healthy individuals and in other non-autoimmune conditions.
- ENA (extractable nuclear antigens) are a group of proteins which, as the name suggests, are extracted from the cell nucleus. As opposed to ANA, they are more specific and are able to pinpoint the antigens for the autoantibodies. In this chapter, we aim to discuss the principle, laboratory techniques, various patterns, and interpretation of ANA testing.

3.2 Methods of Testing ANA

3.2.1 Immunofluorescence

- This is the most reliable and widely used technique for antinuclear antibody testing. It works on the principle of indirect immunofluorescence.
- Serum of patients containing antibodies to nuclear antigens (ANAs) is allowed to react with standard cells called substrate.
- Historically, the rat liver cells were used for ANA assay. However, with advances in technology related to cell cultures, Hep2 cells are used for ANA detection [2].
- Use of Hep-2 cell lines has reduced the chances of ANA negative lupus to <1%.
- If ANAs are present in the patient sera, it binds with the substrate. As the first antibody from patient's sera is not conjugated with any marker, the antigen antibody reaction cannot be detected. For detecting the presence of the antibodies, another anti-human antibody conjugated with fluorescent dye is used (Fig. 3.1).

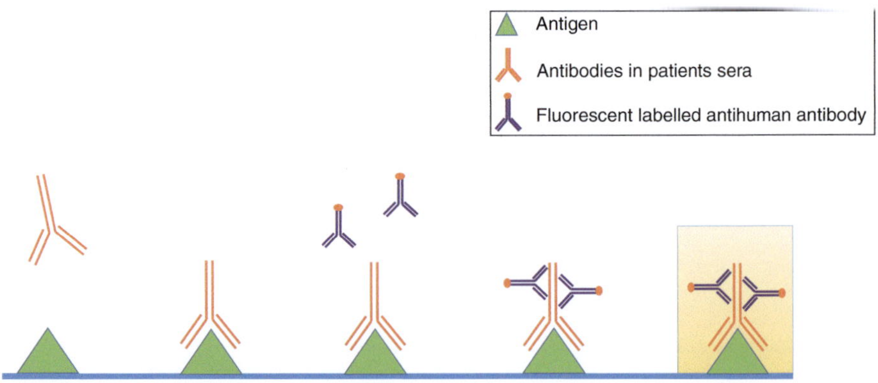

Fig. 3.1 Principle of indirect immunoflourescence

The second conjugated antibody will bind the pathogenic antibodies, and their presence can be detected using a fluorescent microscope.

3.2.2 Enzyme Linked Immunosorbent Assay (ELISA)

- This is also a very sensitive technique used to measure autoantibodies.
- The purified substrate antigens are pre-coated on the well of a polystyrene plate. A patient serum is added to the well, allowed to incubate. Labelled antibody against the human antibody is then added, and the level of the antinuclear antibodies is ascertained on measuring the absorbance of the labelled antibody.
- This technique is used to ascertain levels.

Table 3.1 summarizes the difference between immunofluorescence and ELISA-based assay for ANA [3].

Despite the technical limitations of immunofluorescence, it is recommended as the primary screening technique. ELISA is better suited for identifying the antigen present once the ANA is positive.

3.2.3 Immunoblot Assays

- This is a specialized ELISA technique which is commonly used to ascertain the ENAs.
- It consists of a nitrocellulose strip where common nuclear autoantigens are fixed according to their molecular weight. When the serum is incubated with the strip, a black line appears on the nitrocellulose strip. The autoantigen against which antibodies are produced can be identified on the basis of the location of the line on the strip [4].

Table 3.1 Difference between immunofluorescence and ELISA-based assay for ANA

ANA by indirect immunofluorescence (IIF)	ANA by ELISA
Cumbersome and operator-dependent technique	Standard ELISA kits available. It can be easily automated to run thousands of samples
Substrates (Hep2 cells) have thousands of potential nuclear autoantigens. More sensitive	8–10 purified antigens coated in well are used as substrate Less sensitive
Less chances of false positivity	More chances of false positivity
Information of the pattern of ANA is obtained. It has some clinical significance	Level of autoantibody can be quantitatively obtained. It has no clinical significance

3.3 ANA Patterns and Interpretation

- ANA testing can reveal a variety of distinct patterns of fluorescence, which can provide important clues about the underlying autoimmune disease [5]. In total at least 27 patterns of ANA have been described. The most common patterns are homogeneous, speckled, nucleolar, centromere, and cytoplasmic (Figs. 3.2 and 3.3) (Table 3.2).

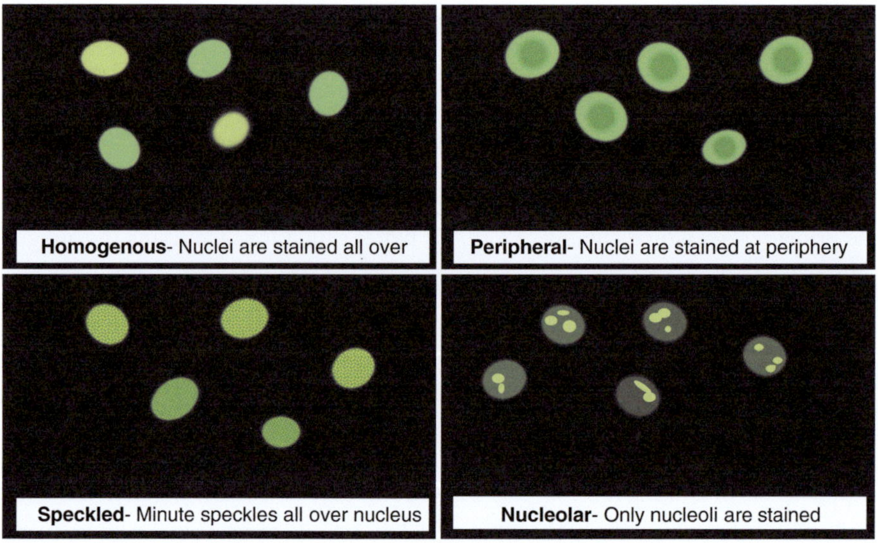

Fig. 3.2 Most common patterns of ANA on Immunofluorescence

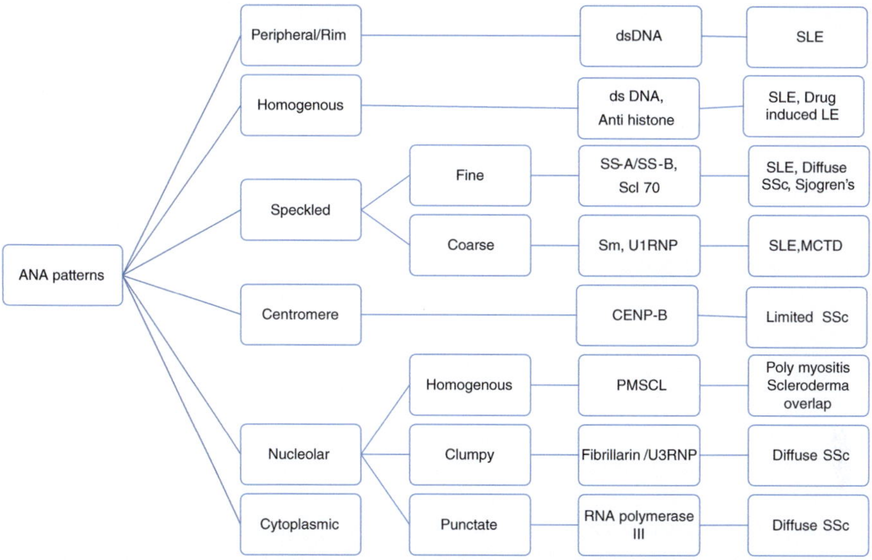

Fig. 3.3 Various patterns of ANA. *SLE* systemic lupus erythematosus, *SSc* systemic sclerosis, *MCTD* mixed connective tissue disease

Table 3.2 Various patterns of ANA

Pattern	Description	Disease
Homogenous	Diffuse distribution of fluorescence throughout the nucleus	Systemic lupus erythematosus May be seen in other AICTDs also
Peripheral/rim	Fluorescence at the periphery of nucleus	Systemic lupus erythematosus
Speckled	Small, discrete foci of fluorescence	Systemic lupus erythematosus Sjogren's syndrome Mixed connective tissue disease
Nucleolar	Bright fluorescence in the nucleolus which is the region responsible for ribosome synthesis	Diffuse cutaneous systemic sclerosis Polymyositis/dermatomyositis
Centromere	Presence of fluorescence around the centromeres of chromosomes	Limited cutaneous systemic sclerosis
Cytoplasmic	Presence of fluorescence in the cytoplasm of cells	Nonspecific pattern Can be seen in non-autoimmune diseases also

Table 3.3 Prevalence of ANA in normal population

Age	Prevalence (%)
5–10 years	3
10–30 years	10–15
30–50 years	10–30
>50 years	15–40

3.4 Titer of ANA

- ANA titers are reported in the dilution at which the sera were tested. Sometimes serial dilution of ANA is required to ascertain the highest dilution at which ANA is positive. The higher the dilution, the higher the concentration of ANA.
- The level after which ANA is considered positive varies among laboratories, but the general consensus regarding level above which ANA is considered to be clinically significant is **>1:160**.
- ANA can be positive even in normal healthy individuals (Table 3.3) and among first-degree relative of a SLE patient [6].

3.5 Clinical Significance of ANAs

- They serve as a valuable screening tool and guide further investigations for the diagnosis and management of autoimmune diseases [7].
- However, it is essential to note that ANA testing alone is not sufficient for a definitive diagnosis of AICTD. While ANA testing is sensitive, it lacks specificity.
- False-positive ANA results can occur in certain infections, chronic liver diseases, malignancies, and during pregnancy. False-negative ANA results can also occur, particularly in some cases of early-stage autoimmune diseases.
- In patients with nonspecific complaints suggestive of AICTD and a positive ANA, it is wise to do **anti DFS 70** antibodies. If this is positive, it is a negative predictor for development of any AICTD.

Therefore, ANA testing should be interpreted alongside the patient's clinical history, physical examination, and other diagnostic tests (Table 3.4).

Table 3.4 Prevalence of ANA in various autoimmune diseases

Diseases where ANA positivity is a mandatory criteria	
Drug-induced lupus	100%
Autoimmune hepatitis	100%
Mixed connective tissue disease	100%
Disease where ANA is useful for diagnosis	
Systemic lupus erythematosus	>98%
Systemic sclerosis	>95%
Polymyositis/dermatomyositis	40–60%
Primary Sjogren's syndrome	40–60%
Disease where ANA is positive as an association	
Rheumatoid arthritis	30–50%
Thyroid disease	30–50%
Immune thrombocytopenia	10–30%
Infections	Wide variations
Fibromyalgia	15–25%

3.6 Importance of ANA in Prognosis and Monitoring

ANA positivity has prognostic significance in Juvenile Idiopathic Arthritis and severity of disease in patients with Raynaud's phenomenon. In other AICTDs, a significant correlation has not yet been established [8].

3.7 Clinical Correlation of ENAs and Clinical Significance

Various ENA have been shown to be associated with specific manifestations of autoimmune diseases as shown in Table 3.5 [9].

Table 3.5 Prevalence of various ENA in autoimmune diseases and their clinical correlation

Antigen	Disease association with prevalence (%)	Clinical significance
SLE		
Nucleosomes	50–90%	Early marker
Ds-DNA	40–90%	Levels correlate with lupus nephritis
Histones	Drug-induced LE (50–90%)	Also in RA, SLE, SSc with pulmonary fibrosis
Sm	20–40%	Specific for SLE
rRNP	30–40%	Neuropsychiatric LE
U1RNP	MCTD (100%), SLE (30–70%)	Presence of U1RNP in absence of other ENA confirms MCTD, otherwise overlaps with DM/SSc
ssDNA	70%	Possible risk of SLE in DLE patients; DM/PM; SSc; morphea
SSA/Ro	50%	SCLE, neonatal LE/congenital heart block; photosensitivity; associated with vasculitis; SCLE-SjS overlap
SSB/La	20%	SCLE; SCLE-SjS overlap
Sjogren's syndrome		
SSA/Ro	Sjogren's disease (40–95%)	May precede diagnosis of SS
SSB/La	Sjogren's disease (40–95%)	May precede diagnosis of SS
Systemic sclerosis		
DNA topoisomerase 1 (Scl 70)	Diffuse cutaneous SSc (60%)	Pulmonary fibrosis, severe digital vasculopathy, scleroderma renal crisis, poor prognosis (highest mortality)
RNA polymerase III	Diffuse cutaneous SSc (45%)	Correlates with extent of skin involvement; scleroderma renal crisis, malignancy association
Centromere (CENP-B)	Limited cutaneous SSc (80%), CREST	Pulmonary artery hypertension, severe gastrointestinal disease
Fibrillarin (U3RNP)	Diffuse cutaneous SSc (5%)	Internal organ involvement, pulmonary artery hypertension, scleroderma renal crisis
Ku	2%	Severe muscle and joint disease, overlap with DM
Polymyositis-scleroderma (pm-Scl)	5% patients with SSc Polymyositis-scleroderma overlap (33%)	Myositis, interstitial lung disease, arthritis
Dermatomyositis		
p 155	DM (20–30%)	CADM, increased malignancy risk, mucosal involvement, poikiloderma, extensive cutaneous involvement
Mi-2	Dermatomyositis (15%)	Specific for DM; cutaneous features
Jo-1	Polymyositis (23–36%)	Antisynthetase syndrome
PL-7	Idiopathic myositis (2–3%)	Antisynthetase syndrome

(continued)

Table 3.5 (continued)

Antigen	Disease association with prevalence (%)	Clinical significance
PL-12	Idiopathic myositis (2–3%)	Antisynthetase syndrome
SRP	Polymyositis (5% and 18% in Jo-1 negative patients)	Fulminant DM/PM, cardiac involvement
MDA 5	DM (10–45%)	CADM, ILD, vasculopathic cutaneous ulcers, oral ulcers, tender palmar papules
NXP 2	DM(1–15% adults; 20% juvenile)	Malignancy association (adults), calcinosis, and severe myositis (juvenile)
PCNA	SLE (03%)	

3.8 Conclusion

Detection and interpretation of antinuclear antibodies (ANAs) play a vital role in the diagnosis and management of autoimmune diseases. ANA testing serves as a valuable screening tool, aiding healthcare providers in identifying patients who may have underlying autoimmune conditions, but it should not be relied upon as a standalone diagnostic tool, as it lacks specificity and can be positive in non-autoimmune conditions. The various patterns observed in ANA testing, such as homogeneous, speckled, nucleolar, centromere, and cytoplasmic, provide important clues to the specific autoimmune diseases involved. Although these patterns are associated with certain diseases, they are not pathognomonic and must be evaluated in conjunction with clinical history, physical examination, and additional diagnostic tests for accurate diagnosis. While ANA testing has limitations, it remains valuable in monitoring disease activity and treatment response in autoimmune diseases. As the field of ANA research continues to evolve, future advancements in ANA testing methods and interpretation may enhance diagnostic accuracy and improve patient outcomes. Additionally, a deeper understanding of the pathogenesis and clinical significance of ANAs may lead to the development of targeted therapies and personalized medicine approaches for autoimmune diseases.

References

1. Agmon-Levin N, Damoiseaux J, Kallenberg C, et al. International recommendations for the assessment of autoantibodies to cellular antigens referred to as anti-nuclear antibodies. Ann Rheum Dis. 2014;73:17–23.
2. Tebo AE, Schmidt RL, Kadkhoda K, et al. The antinuclear antibody HEp-2 indirect immunofluorescence assay: a survey of laboratory performance, pattern recognition and interpretation. Autoimmune Highlights. 2021;12:4.
3. Rondeel JM. Immunofluorescence versus ELISA for the detection of antinuclear antigens. Expert Rev Mol Diagnosis. 2002;2(3):226–32.
4. Capín NG, Rodriguez MR, Lavalle CM, et al. Immunoblot assay for detection of autoantibodies in autoimmune disease. J Clin Lab Anal. 1992;6(5):319–23.

5. Mariz HA, Sato EI, Barbosa SH, et al. Pattern on the antinuclear antibody-HEp-2 test is a critical parameter for discriminating anti- nuclear antibody-positive healthy individuals and patients with autoimmune rheumatic diseases. Arthritis Rheum. 2011;63:191–200.
6. Grygiel-Górniak B, Rogacka N, Puszczewicz M. Antinuclear antibodies in healthy people and non-rheumatic diseases – diagnostic and clinical implications. Reumatologia. 2018;56(4):243–8.
7. Kavanaugh A, Tomar R, Reveille J, et al. Guidelines for clinical use of the antinuclear antibody test and tests for specific autoantibodies to nuclear antigens, American College of Pathologists. Arch Pathol Lab Med. 2000;124:71–81.
8. Ravelli A, Felici E, Magni-Manzoni S, et al. Patients with antinuclear antibody-positive juvenile idiopathic arthritis constitutes a homogeneous subgroup irrespective of the course of joint disease. Arthritis Rheum. 2005;52(3):826–32.
9. Selmi C, Ceribelli A, Generali E, et al. Serum antinuclear and extractable nuclear antigen antibody prevalence and associated morbidity and mortality in the general population over 15 years. Autoimmun Rev. 2016;15(2):162–6.

Investigations

4

Pooja Agarwal and Kalgi Baxi

Abstract

Autoimmune connective tissue diseases (AICTDs) are a heterogeneous group of systemic disorders and usually require in-depth investigations. While some investigations are mandatory at baseline to know the extent of involvement, others are done later to further confirm the disease burden. The significance and implications of various haematological, histopathological and radiological investigations are highlighted in this chapter.

Keywords

Haematological · Urine analysis · Histopathology · Radiology

4.1 Introduction

The most daunting dilemma that a dermatologist faces when coming across a patient with autoimmune connective tissue disease (AICTDs) is the investigation part. A sound understanding of rationale is essential before subjecting the patient to a battery of tests to prevent unnecessary burden on the patient. Details of antinuclear antibodies (ANA) and extractable nuclear antigens (ENA) have been discussed in Chap. 3, and the current chapter will focus on developing an approach towards investigating a patient with autoimmune connective tissue disease. The figure (Fig. 4.1) below outlines a simplified clinical approach for patients presenting with clinical signs and symptoms of autoimmune connective tissue diseases.

P. Agarwal · K. Baxi (✉)
Department of Skin & VD, SVPIMSR, Smt NHL Municipal Medical College, Ahmedabad, Gujarat, India

P. Agarwal et al. (eds.), *Dermatologist's Handbook of Autoimmune Connective Tissue Diseases*, https://doi.org/10.1007/978-981-95-0524-1_4

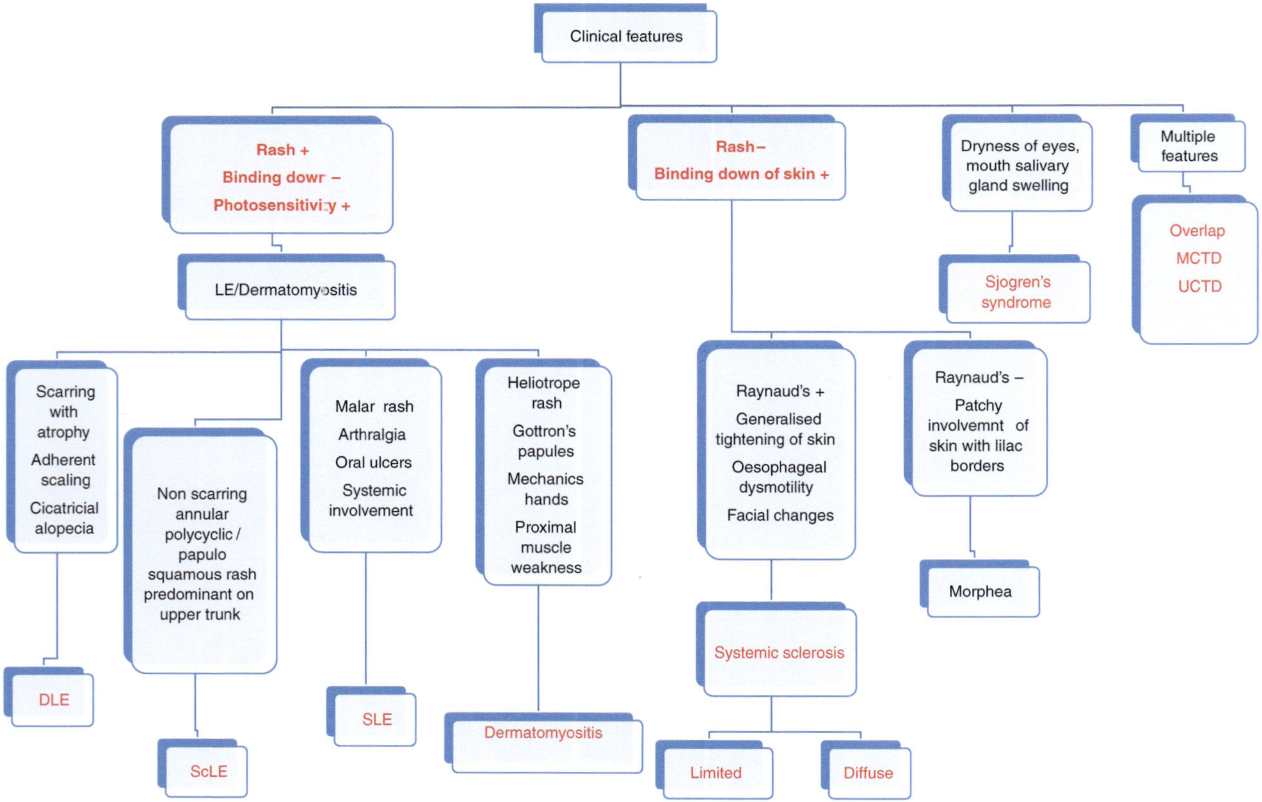

Fig. 4.1 Flowchart illustrating clinical approach for diagnosis of autoimmune connective tissue disorders. *DLE* discoid lupus erythematosus, *ScLe* subacute cutaneous lupus erythematosus, *SLE* systemic lupus erythematosus, *MCTD* mixed connective tissue disease, *UCTD* undifferentiated connective tissue disease

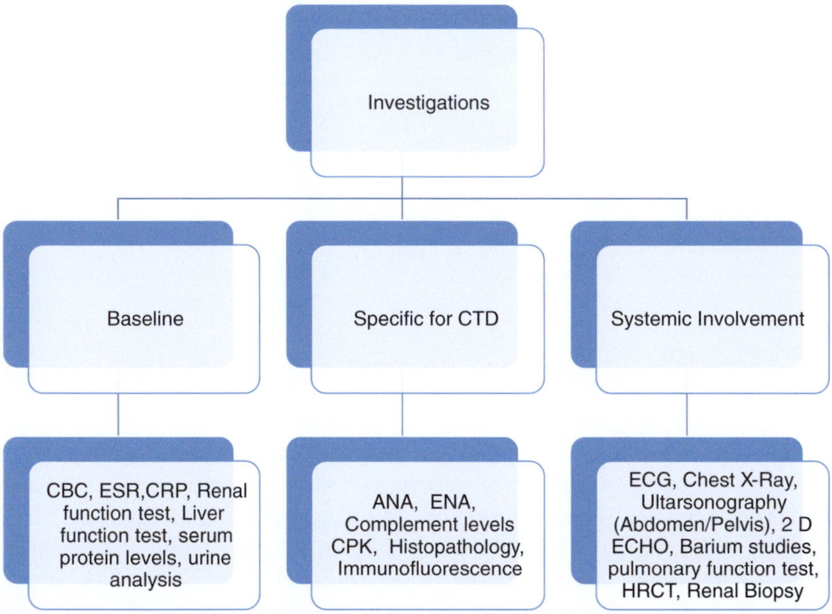

Fig. 4.2 Illustration of investigation in AICTDs

Investigations: A Practical Approach

The investigations can be broadly classified as baseline laboratory investigations, investigations which help in diagnosing the disease specifically, and special investigations which help in assessing the organ involvement (Fig. 4.2).

4.2 Baseline Laboratory Investigations

4.2.1 Haematological

They form important part in initial workup of the patient and establish a baseline for assessing the progression of disease or treatment response. These help in the overall assessment of the patient's condition. Some of these provide a clue to an underlying systemic involvement also which may not be apparent clinically in initial stages.

- **Complete blood count (CBC):** This includes the haemoglobin levels, total leucocyte counts, differential counts, RBC indices and peripheral smear. Various abnormalities which can be seen in the CBC are listed in Table 4.1.
- **Erythrocyte sedimentation rate (ESR)**: A commonly overlooked investigation is ESR which gives us the earliest clue regarding the chronic nature of the disease. It is raised in SLE and less commonly in systemic sclerosis.

Table 4.1 Various abnormalities in complete blood count in various AICTDs

Anaemia (Hb < 10 g)	Leucopaenia (total count<4000)	Thrombocytopaenia (platelet count<100,000)
In SLE Chronic disease Renal insufficiency Haemolysis Iron deficiency In systemic sclerosis Inadequate food intake Malabsorption Renal involvement GI bleed	Bone marrow suppression Due to disease Due to therapy	Bone marrow suppression Associated immune thrombocytopenic purpura

- **C-Reactive Protein (CRP):** CRP is an acute phase reactant secreted by the hepatocytes, and along with ESR it serves as an important biomarker for active inflammatory state. Though levels of CRP generally correlate with the disease activity in the majority of inflammatory diseases, CRP is an unreliable biomarker for systemic lupus erythematosus (SLE), inflammatory myopathies, primary Sjogren and other type 1 interferon alpha driven diseases. Interpretation of CRP levels in background of AICTDs should be cautious, as multiple confounding factors exist such as the following:
  - History of ongoing treatment with multiple immunosuppressant drugs makes the patients more prone to acquiring infections. High-dose corticosteroids and JAK inhibitors in particular interfere with IL-6 signalling and in turn CRP levels.
  - Presence of malignancies mimicking AICTDs, as well as increased incidence of certain cancers with rheumatic diseases, can affect the CRP levels.
- **Liver Function Tests** [1].

Liver involvement in AICTDs can be:

(a) Autoimmune
(b) Coexistent non-immune hepatopathy (e.g. drug related, thrombotic microangiopathy, infectious hepatitis)
(c) Disease-specific parenchymal involvement, e.g. lupoid hepatitis.
Autoimmune hepatitis is characterised by elevated transaminases, increased IgG levels, presence of autoantibodies and histopathological changes consistent with interface hepatitis. Early diagnosis of autoimmune hepatitis is important as it has a propensity to progress to liver cirrhosis. Liver biopsy remains the investigation of choice for assessing liver inflammation and fibrosis. Red blood cell

distribution width (RDW) and prothrombin time (PT) have been considered and are under further research as surrogate markers of advanced liver inflammation.

- **Renal function test**: It includes blood urea, serum creatinine and electrolytes. Both SLE and systemic sclerosis (SSc) have early renal involvement; hence regular monitoring is essential. Frequent checks (every 3 months) for creatinine, proteinuria, anti-dsDNA antibodies, and complement (C3, C4) are recommended for monitoring of lupus nephritis.
- **Serum protein levels**: Low albumin levels are seen in case of lupus nephritis due to proteinuria. While in systemic sclerosis, hypoalbuminemia may be due to malnutrition and malabsorption.

4.2.2 Urine Analysis [2–4]

As the renal involvement is a common feature in most connective tissue diseases, urine examination forms an integral part of the workup. It encompasses the basic urine analysis on spot as well as after collecting the urine for 24 hours (Table 4.2).

Urine routine and microscopy findings in case of systemic lupus erythematosus reflect the severity and grade of lupus nephritis as summarised in Table 4.3.

Table 4.2 Urine analysis in SLE and SSc

SLE	Systemic sclerosis
24-hour urinary protein: Gold standard for accurate measurement of proteinuria >0.5 g/day	Mild proteinuria and haematuria with granular casts are suggestive of scleroderma renal crisis in context of increasing serum creatinine and hypertension Proteinuria >1 g/day in SSc is uncommon and suggests an underlying glomerular disorder. In regard to SSc, epidemiological studies have identified proteinuria as a risk factor for increased mortality
Spot urine protein/creatinine ratio; should normally be less than 0.3	
Urinary casts: Red blood cell casts: Suggestive of lupus nephritis Granular and waxy casts: Suggests grade 4 and grade 5 lupus nephritis	
American college rheumatology definition of lupus nephritis: Lupus nephritis is defined as PERSISTENT PROTEINURIA>0.5 g/d or greater than 3+ on dipstick and /or cellular casts including red blood cells, haemoglobin, granular, tubular or mixed For monitoring 3 monthly proteinuria assessment: Preferably via 24-hour urine collection Alternatively, the protein/creatinine ratio in a morning urine sample	

Table 4.3 Urine analysis in various lupus nephritis

Urine routine and microscopy findings	Corresponding clinical and serological changes	Corresponding grade of lupus nephritis
Normal	–	Incidental findings suggestive of minimal mesangial nephritis
Microhaematuria or non-nephrotic proteinuria	–	Proliferative mesangial lupus nephritis; podocytopathy must also be ruled out
Proteinuria and haematuria	Raised serum creatinine; clinical signs and symptoms s/o hypertension, nephrotic syndrome Elevated anti-dsDNA titres, presence of hypocomplementemia	Focal and diffuse (class 3 and class 4) lupus nephritis Especially with class 4 nephritis
Nephrotic range proteinuria No haematuria or urinary sediment	Normal renal parameters; nephrotic syndrome +/–	Class 5: Membranous lupus nephritis; immunological activity is negligible
	Progressively worsening serum urea, creatinine values and deteriorated renal function	Class 6: Sclerosing lupus nephritis

4.3 Investigations Specific for the Connective Tissue Diseases [5–11]

These investigations form the next step of the ladder and help in reaching towards the definitive diagnosis. However, as the spectrum of the autoimmune connective is so vast, it may not always be possible to label the patient under one specific disease. In such cases, it is important to follow up the patient with regular screening as later one or the other serologic markers for the disease may become evident. Even when the conclusive diagnosis has been made, it is important to repeat some of these investigations on a regular basis.

4.3.1 Haematological

ANA, ENA, serum complement levels, serum creatine phosphokinase levels
Details of the antinuclear and extractable antigens and their significance have been discussed in the previous chapter.

- **Anti-nuclear antibodies**: This forms the first step of labelling a patient as having an autoimmune CTD. Detection of ANA by indirect immunofluorescence method is better than ELISA technique to overcome any false-negative results.
- **Extractable nuclear antigens**: The next step towards reaching a more specific diagnosis amongst the CTD is to order the ENA or sometimes referred to as ANA immunoblot.

- **Serum complement levels:**
  Activation of the complement cascade is one of key aspects in the pathogenesis of AICTDs. Though multiple by-products of the complement pathways have been found to have pathological significance in the diagnosis, prognosis, severity and organ damage associated with the disease, practically, levels of serum C3 and C4 are assessed in clinical practice. Table 4.4 outlines the interpretation and significance of complement levels associated with various AICTDs.
- **Serum CPK** [12–20]

Table 4.4 Interpretation of serum complement levels in AICTDs

Disease	Serum complement profile	Interpretation	Newer complement biomarkers
Systemic lupus erythematosus	Decreased C3 and/or C4 levels	Part of diagnostic criteria SLICC-2012 as well as 2019 EULAR/ACR criteria The frequency of hypocomplementemia at diagnosis of SLE is 50–89% Organ involvement: Positive association with lupus nephritis, autoimmune haemolytic anaemia and thrombocytopenia, cutaneous involvement, and arthritis Disease activity: Non-specific correlation	**Serum C1q**: Decreased levels associated with higher disease activity **Split products of C3,C4**: Cleavage products of C3,C4 (iC3b and C4d) are better biomarkers; however laboratory assays to quantify them are underway *Cell-bound complement activation product (CB-CAP)*: More sensitive in assessing disease activity. CB-CAP bound to platelets is useful in predicting thrombotic and other vascular events
Systemic sclerosis	Low	Decreased levels have been linked, to overlapping conditions and myositis	Increased levels of complement degradation products have been associated with diffuse systemic sclerosis and interstitial lung disease
Dermatomyositis	Low	C4 hypocomplementemia has been associated with malignancy risk in dermatomyositis	Tissue deposited and cell bound complement fragments, e.g. higher E-C4d levels are markers of chronic complement activation
Mixed connective tissue disease	Low	Complement activation in MCTD by anti U1RNP antibodies can induce non-erosive arthritis, myositis and interstitial lung disease in MCTD patients	–

Serum CPK Levels in Systemic Lupus Erythematosus

Values of creatine phosphokinase are generally low in patients of SLE; hence even a slight elevation above the normal values is considered clinically significant for diagnosis of SLE myositis. LE myopathy has been defined as:

1. Elevated creatine kinase.
2. Documented muscle oedema on MRI.
3. Myopathic electromyography.
4. And/or myopathic muscle biopsy features (including myofiber necrosis, perifascicular atrophy, perivascular inflammation, primary lymphocytic inflammation).

Moreover elevation of serum CK levels could also be a marker for SLE-dermatomyositis overlap syndrome, which can be diagnosed by presence of myositis-specific and myositis-associated antibodies. An important and often under-recognised cause of elevated muscle enzymes in SLE is chronic antimalarial therapy, albeit seldom evolving into full-fledged clinical myopathy. Conversely, presence of proximal muscle weakness in setting of normal CK levels should raise a suspicion of glucocorticoid-induced myopathy in relevant case scenario.

Serum CPK Levels in Systemic Sclerosis

Serum CPK values have not been validated for SSc, although they have been found to negatively correlate with muscle strength. However a significant number of patients with objective evidence of muscle involvement have a normal CK level. For diagnosis of SSc-specific myositis, a combination of serum CPK levels and aldolase is more sensitive. More recently, a phenotype of SSc-specific myositis has been termed as "Minimal myositis with capillary pathology" (MMCP), which is distinctly different from myositis-SSc overlap and is recognised by a very mild elevation of serum CK levels and histopathological evidence of capillary enlargement in muscle biopsy with mild inflammatory infiltration.

Serum CPK Levels in Dermatomyositis

About 90% of patients with dermatomyositis present with symmetrical proximal muscle weakness and elevated creatine kinase levels, which can be as high as 50 times the upper normal limit. Subsets of patients with clinically amyopathic dermatomyositis however present with normal CK levels and hence present a diagnostic challenge. This subset is usually associated with anti-MDA5 antibody. Serum creatine kinase (CK) level is the most sensitive but not specific indicator for dermatomyositis. The CK level does not usually correlate with the severity of the symptoms among different patients. However its value lies in reflecting changes in disease activity in an individual patient.

Serum CPK Levels in MCTD

Approximately 72% of patients with MCTD present with a subclinical increase in muscle enzyme levels. However only a meagre 2–3% of these present with clinical signs and symptoms of myositis in the initial stages. The myositis associated with MCTD is generally milder than the inflammatory myositis of dermatomyositis.

4.3.2 Histopathology and Immunofluorescence [21, 22]

SLE

Histopathology plays a major role in the diagnosis of cutaneous lupus and reflects the real-time changes occurring in the skin. The classification of cutaneous lesions into LE-specific and LE-nonspecific is based on pathognomic histological changes. Furthermore, the presence of these changes at various levels within the skin defines various subsets of cutaneous LE (Fig. 4.3, Table 4.5).

Systemic Sclerosis (Table 4.6)

- Histopathology is generally not required for the diagnosis of systemic sclerosis; its role mainly lies in case of clinical dilemma to rule out scleroderma-like syndromes.

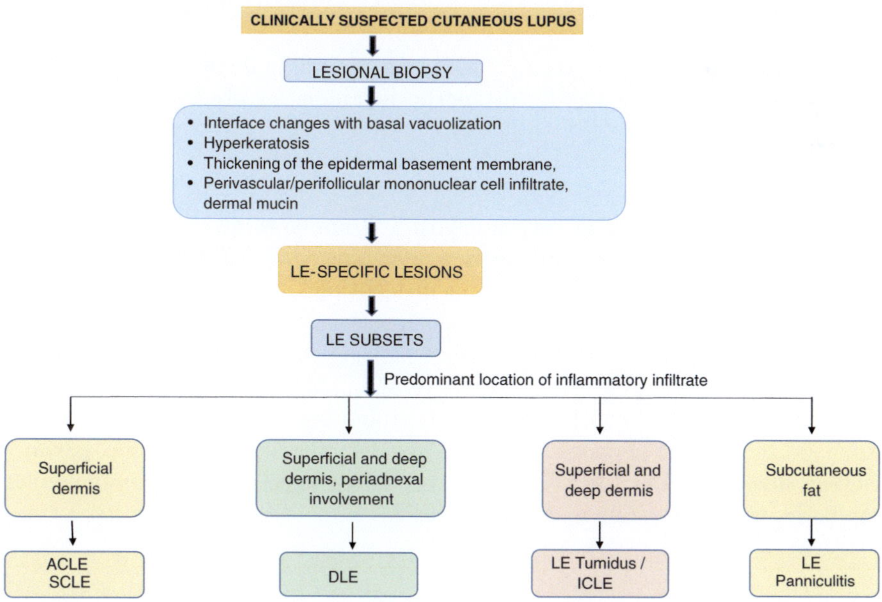

Fig. 4.3 LE subsets. *ACLE* acute cutaneous lupus erythematosus, *SCLE* subacute cutaneous lupus erythematosus, *DLE* discoid lupus erythematosus, *ICLE* intermittent cutaneous lupus erythematosus

Table 4.5 Histopathological findings in various subsets of lupus erythematosus

	DLE	SCLE	SLE
Follicular plugging	+++	–	–
Thickened BM	+++	+	+
Periappendageal inflammation	+++	+	–
Pilosebaceous atrophy	+++	–	–
Perivascular infiltrate	+	+	++
Oedema of dermis	++	+++	+
Inflammatory infiltrate	+++	++	+
Involvement of s/c fat	–	–	+++

Table 4.6 Histological changes in early and late stage of systemic sclerosis

Early inflammatory stage	Late sclerotic stage
Moderately severe inflammatory cell infiltrate, predominately lymphoplasmacytic, in between collagen bundles and around blood vessels. Infiltrate may extend into subcutaneous fat and project around eccrine glands Wavy collagen fibres within the reticular dermis and subcutaneous fat Vascular changes in the form of endothelial swelling	Inflammatory infiltrate has disappeared Collagen is closely packed and eccrine glands appear atrophic or absent. Collagen may replace fat cells in the subcutaneous tissue Few blood vessels are noted here; they often have fibrotic walls with narrowed lumen

- It is important that the biopsy specimen includes **adequate amount of subcutaneous tissue**, since most of the diagnostic alterations are observed there.

Dermatomyositis

Cutaneous histopathology of dermatomyositis is **non-specific** and resembles systemic lupus erythematosus with interface dermatitis, vacuolar degeneration of the stratum basale and significant dermal mucin deposition. In addition, **vasculopathic changes** including endothelial injury, vascular ectasia, vessel thickening and extravasation of red blood cells are also an important histopathology finding in a subset of patients. **Gottron's papules** show acanthosis and mild papillomatosis.

Muscle histopathology: Histopathological findings of muscle biopsy are characteristic and include perivascular and perimysial inflammatory infiltrate, **perifascicular atrophy (HALLMARK)** and endothelial hyperplasia of intramuscular capillaries with a reduction in capillary density.

4.3.3 Direct Immunofluorescence (DIF)

Direct immunofluorescence is useful for the detection of tissue-bound autoantibodies and plays an important role in confirmatory diagnosis of autoimmune connective tissue diseases, especially systemic lupus erythematosus.

Table 4.7 Pattern of deposition of immunoreactant on DIF

Pattern of deposition of immunoreactants on DIF
Continuous band of granular deposition at DEJ; higher magnification shows various patterns such as: Linear Homogenous: In chronic or atrophic lesions Fibrillar Stippled (most common) Shaggy Lumpy Thready
Discontinuous band: Less specific for lupus; seen in: Healthy exposed skin Rosacea Actinic keratosis Polymorphic light eruption
Immunoreactants: Commonest component deposited: Complement C3 Commonest immunoglobulin class: IgM IgG, IgA may also be present; so called as the "full-house" pattern Clinical correlation: Various studies have concluded that SLE patients with positive DIF and > 1 immunoreactant on lesional and nonlesional skin have a higher immunological profile and increased SLE disease activity.

Table 4.8 Lupus band test in various lupus subtypes

	Lesional skin	Nonlesional, sun-exposed skin	Nonlesional, non-sun-exposed skin
SLE	++	++	++
SCLE	+	+/–	–
DLE	+	–	–

- **Lupus band test:** Presence of one or more immunoreactants (IgG, IgM, IgA and complement components) (Tables 4.7 and 4.8) in a linear configuration at the dermo-epidermal junction along with the basement membrane is considered as a positive lupus band test.

  DIF is not routinely performed in other connective tissue diseases.

4.4 Investigations to Rule Out Systemic Complications [23–27]

All the AICTDs are multisystem disorders with significant, often life-threatening complications. Hence a battery of investigations is carried out once the diagnosis of CTD is confirmed to diagnose the extent and severity of internal organ involvement (Table 4.9).

Table 4.9 Investigations for diagnosis of cardiac complications in autoimmune connective tissue diseases

Disease	Timing of performing ECG and 2D echo	ECG findings	2D echo findings
SLE	At the diagnosis	ST-T and T wave changes: Most common Bradyarrhythmia, heart blocks and QT prolongation Structural ECG abnormalities like hypertrophic cardiomyopathy (may be associated with chronic antimalarial therapy) Increased incidence of fragmented QRS complex (f QRS)—Pulmonary hypertension and resulting right and left ventricular dysfunction secondary to PH	Diagnosis of: SLE-related pericarditis, systolic dysfunction, valvular involvement (Libman-sacks endocarditis) and cavity thrombus formation with a good sensitivity. Transesophageal echocardiography may be needed for closer analysis of valve structure and function and is thus more sensitive Myocarditis (especially during LE flare): Global or segmental wall motion abnormalities
Systemic sclerosis	ECG and 2D echo At diagnosis and yearly thereafter if no abnormality detected	An abnormal ECG has historically been shown to be present in 25–75% of SSc patients and is considered an independent predictor of mortality Fragmented QRS complex, Tp-e interval (the interval between the peak and end of the T-wave) are independent predictors of cardiovascular mortality associated with systemic sclerosis Ventricular tachyarrhythmias	For timely decision to perform right heart catheterisation in patients with PAH, 2D echo criteria remain the core guideline; if the tricuspid regurgitant velocity is more than 2.8 m/s, or more than 2.5 m/s in presence of signs or symptoms of PH To detect involvement of myocardium and valvular complex due to myocardial fibrosis

(continued)

Table 4.9 (continued)

Disease	Timing of performing ECG and 2D echo	ECG findings	2D echo findings
Dermatomyositis	ECG at the first visit on diagnosis; subsequent investigations based on personal history, signs and symptoms of cardiac involvement	ECG: ECG abnormalities are common and may include atrial or ventricular premature beats, arrhythmias and bundle branch blocks. The rhythm abnormalities are more often clinically irrelevant	Echocardiography: Important to diagnose myocardial dysfunction; left ventricular diastolic dysfunction being the commonest finding Valvular abnormalities, chamber or septal hypertrophy, global hypokinesia and pulmonary hypertension are the other abnormalities
MCTD	No guidelines exist regarding cardiac assessment in MCTD, as it is not primarily involved very often	–	Baseline assessment for ruling out PAH, and other involvement such as pericarditis, myocarditis, mitral valve prolapse, left ventricular (LV) hypertrophy, LV diastolic dysfunction, conduction abnormalities or coronary atherosclerosis

4.4.1 Electrocardiogram and 2D Echocardiography

Electrocardiogram and 2D echocardiography remain the cornerstone investigations for cardiac involvement.

Various parameters assessed on 2D echocardiography along with tissue Doppler imaging include cardiac chamber size, volumes and movement, wall motion abnormalities, left ventricular ejection fraction, mitral annular plane systolic excursion (MAPSE), tricuspid annular plane systolic excursion (TAPSE) and mitral and tricuspid regurgitation velocity.

4.4.2 Radiological Investigations [28–34]

4.4.2.1 Chest X-Ray (Table 4.10)

4.4.2.2 High-Resolution Computed Tomography (HRCT)

HRCT is considered as a gold standard investigation in the diagnosis of interstitial lung disease in systemic sclerosis, dermatomyositis (anti-synthetase syndrome) and mixed connective tissue disease. Connective tissue disease associated interstitial

Table 4.10 Chest X-ray finding in various AICTDs

SLE	Systemic sclerosis	Dermatomyositis
Blunting of costophrenic angle: Pleural effusion Elevated right hemidiaphragm without any clear parenchymal disease: Shrinking lung syndrome	Interstitial lung disease (HRCT serves as a better diagnostic tool)	ILD: Antisynthetase syndrome Soft tissue calcifications: In case of generalised calcinosis cutis Malignancy and metastasis screening: Paraneoplastic dermatomyositis

lung disease, often abbreviated as "CTD-ILD", is associated with classical pathognomic radiological patterns, which are:

- Nonspecific interstitial pneumonia (NSIP).
- Usual interstitial pneumonia (UIP).
- Lymphoid interstitial pneumonia (LIP).
- Organizing pneumonia (OP).
- Diffuse alveolar damage (DAD).
- Diffuse alveolar haemorrhage (DAH).

Other classical presentation of CTD-ILD on HRCT may be focal or a diffuse pulmonary abnormality, especially at the periphery of the lung, such as reticulation, ground-glass opacities (GGOs) (which refer to focal or diffuse veil-like opacification of the lung) and nodules.

HRCT serves as an effective tool to diagnose, assess and judge the severity of lung involvement as well as to predict prognosis especially in systemic sclerosis and antisynthetase syndrome.

4.4.2.3 Ultrasonography

The extent of multisystemic involvement in autoimmune connective tissue diseases necessitates periodic investigations and imaging. Ultrasonography is one of the safest "radiations"-free imaging techniques.

4.4.2.3.1 SLE

USG has been used in SLE with musculoskeletal involvement to diagnose synovivits, tenosynovitis and synovial effusion, especially in patients with arthralgia but without clinical synovitis, and for the early identification of bone erosions. Ultrasound studies have shown that 27% of lupus patients with inflammatory joint pain had subclinical synovitis or tenosynovitis. It is also used to diagnose serositis, especially pleuritis and peritoneal inflammation and ascites associated with SLE.

4.4.2.3.2 Systemic Sclerosis

Skin evaluation: High-resolution USG has recently been evaluated for assessment of skin in patients with both localised and diffuse SSc. Majority of the researchers have used an 18–32 MHz probe for a satisfactory resolution of various skin layers.

Advantages of HRUS over clinically evaluated modified Rodnan skin scoring include the following:

- Early detection of skin involvement.
- Evaluation of dermal thickness which correlates with the clinical phase of the disease (oedematous, fibrotic or atrophic).
- Drastically reduced inter- and intra-observer variability as compared to MRSS, reproducibility and an ability for disease staging, for prognosis.

The role of HRUS is also being investigated in the assessment of digital ulcers. Ultrasound is feasible for evaluating various ulcer types, including those on the fingertips, overlying the extensor (dorsal) aspects of the hands and underlying subcutaneous calcinosis. HRUS may also provide new insights into the pathogenesis of development of digital ulcers.

4.4.2.4 Barium Studies

Barium swallow, barium meal and barium meal follow through are usually carried out in patients with systemic sclerosis for assessing the involvement of gastrointestinal tract (Table 4.11).

4.4.2.5 Magnetic Resonance Imaging (MRI)

The various findings are summarised in Table 4.12.

Table 4.11 Barium study findings

Organ involved	Findings on barium studies
Oesophagus: Reflux, dysmotility	Barium swallow reveals a patulous lower oesophageal sphincter and dilatation and aperistalsis predominantly affecting the lower oesophageal sphincter
Stomach: Gastroparesis	Dilated, atonic stomach
Small intestine: Dysmotility	Barium meal follow through: Dilated duodenum and jejunum with loss of duodeno-jejuno junction "Accordion sign"/hide bound bowel sign: Pathognomic sign; presence of >7 jejunal folds (normal 4–7 folds) in context of jejunal dilatation gives this characteristic appearance, and it results from bowel fibrosis and atrophy Presence of wide mouthed diverticula on antimesenteric border of the jejunum
Findings on contrast CT	
Pneumatosis cystoides intestinalis: Presence of radiolucent air-filled cysts in the submucosal and subserosal layers in colon and small bowel Dilated colon with loss of haustra; dilatation may be as prominent as Hirschsprung's disease	

Table 4.12 MRI finding of various AICTDs

AICTD	MRI findings
SLE	Early diagnosis of non-erosive polyarthritis: Bone marrow oedema, joint effusion, subtle erosions and capsuloligamentous thickening can be seen Symmetrical, deforming, non-erosive, and reducible arthropathy ("Jaccoud's arthropathy"): MRI is the investigation of choice for the resultant deformities, which are underestimated on the radiographs, owing to their reducible nature For early diagnosis of avascular necrosis in active SLE or concurrent APLA cases
Systemic sclerosis	Soft tissue calcifications, calcinosis cutis, acroosteolysis in long-standing Raynaud's phenomenon
Dermatomyositis	Muscle MRI is a gold standard for choosing biopsy site in a suspected case of polymyositis/dermatomyositis T2 weighted MRI: Widespread but patchy oedema-like changes in affected muscles, with or without associated fasciitis T1 weighted: Identification of late fatty involution of muscles, which is a conspicuous marker of dermatomyositis-induced chronic damage Soft tissue calcifications: Can be tumoural/globular or sheet like Sheet like/exoskeleton type of calcinosis is a classic sign of dermatomyositis, but not specific
MCTD	Radiological signs are very polymorphic and can mimic or be a combination of any of the above-mentioned diseases

Table 4.13 Pulmonary function test parameters in AICTD

PFT parameters	Changes in systemic sclerosis	Changes in dermatomyositis	Changes in mixed connective tissue disease
Forced vital capacity	FVC/DLCO ratio, along with other parameters (see below): Sensitive for screening for PAH	Reduced Marked reduction (<60%), combined with Hamman-rich presentation (acute interstitial pneumonia with fulminant respiratory failure), CADM, older age and acute/subacute onset of ILD, has been found to correlate with poor prognosis	Remains stable for years; declines only in active disease
Total lung capacity	Correlates well with ILD severity	Both TLC and DLCO correlate with disease severity and treatment response	Same as FVC
DLCO	Steady reduction in active ILD; correlates best with disease severity and early prediction of organ damage		Declines early in the course of disease as an early marker of ILD

4.4.3 Pulmonary Function Tests [35–37]

Pulmonary functions tests (Table 4.13) serve as a diagnostic and prognostic modality to evaluate lung damage associated with AICTDs. Even though used extensively in institutes and research, the role of pulmonary function tests for early detection of lung damage in AICTD is limited, in the absence of HRCT.

Currently the most sensitive method to screen SSc patients for PAH is a composite, two-step, algorithm named DETECT. Items considered in this algorithm are:

- FVC%/DLCO% ratio.
- Presence of ACA and telangiectasia.
- Serum level of NT-proBNP.
- Serum urate.
- Presence of right axis deviation on electrocardiogram.

4.4.4 Renal Biopsy [4]

Renal biopsy is a gold standard investigation for the diagnosis, staging, and management of lupus nephritis.

Indications

- Significant proteinuria ($\geq$0.5 g/24 h).
- Haematuria.
- Active urinary sediment.
- Unexplained deterioration in renal function.
- Repeat or second biopsy very rarely indicated in cases where transition to a more severe class or persistent deterioration on standard treatment is observed.

Lupus nephritis has been classified into six classes based on the histopathological, immunological and electron microscopic findings. Apart from these, other pathological changes that may affect the kidney in lupus include tubulointerstitial disease, podocytopathy and vasculitis.

4.5 Screening Investigations for Malignancy in AICTD [38, 39]

The incidence of malignancy associated with AICTDs has been found to be elevated in multiple large, multicentric studies. Although there is no consensus guideline on routine malignancy screening in AICTDs, the presence of certain risk factors warrants screening in addition to the age and sex appropriate guidelines.

In SLE, dermatomyositis, and scleroderma, the incidence of cancer is highest in the early years following diagnosis (3–5 years). A statistically significant association between MCTD and cancer has not yet been reported although anecdotal

Table 4.14 Risk factors and relevant investigations for screening

Disease	Risk factors for increased incidence of cancer	Screening guidelines
SLE	*Chronic immunosuppression (increased risk of cervical carcinoma)	Regular monitoring of complete haemogram LDH levels, if complaints of fever, night sweats and weight loss occur (B symptoms) Annual pap smears for monitoring of cervical intraepithelial neoplasia
Systemic sclerosis	*Presence of anti RNA polymerase III autoantibodies on immunoblot	Complete radiological and clinical screening for cancer at the time of diagnosis (HRCT thorax, abdomen, mammography, prostrate examination) To watch for unexplained dysphagia
Dermatomyositis	Presence of anti-TIF1 gamma and antiNXP2 autoantibodies	Chest, abdomen, pelvic CT and pelvic ultrasound at the time of diagnosis

reports exist. Other risk factors and relevant investigations have been summarised below (Table 4.14).

4.6 Conclusion

Though the list of investigations is exhaustive and beyond scope of this chapter, it summarises investigations for workup of an AICTD case. The reader is advised to corroborate the findings with clinical features and diagnostic workup advised in the individual chapters covering separate entities in this book. This should help a treating dermatologist to interpret and appropriately advise and refer the patients for necessary tests.

References

1. Fang X, Zaman MH, Guo X, Ding H, Xie C, Zhang X, Deng GM. Role of hepatic deposited immunoglobulin G in the pathogenesis of liver damage in systemic lupus erythematosus. Front Immunol. 2018;9:1457.
2. Chrabaszcz M, Małyszko J, Sikora M, Alda-Malicka R, Stochmal A, Matuszkiewicz-Rowinska J, et al. Renal involvement in systemic sclerosis: an update. Kidney Blood Press Res. 2020;45:532–48.
3. Hahn BH, McMahon MA, Wilkinson A, et al. American College of Rheumatology guidelines for screening, treatment, and management of lupus nephritis. Arthritis Care Res (Hoboken). 2012;64:797–808.
4. Ruiz Irastorza G, Espinosa G, Frutos MA, Jiménez Alonso J, Praga M, Pallarés L, Rivera F, Robles Marhuenda Á, Segarra A, Quereda C. Diagnosis and treatment of lupus nephritis. Consensus document from the systemic auto-immune disease group (GEAS) of the Spanish Society of Internal Medicine (SEMI) and the Spanish Society of Nephrology (SEN). Nefrología (English Edition). 2012;32:1–35.

5. Pons-Estel GJ, Ugarte-Gil MF, Harvey GB, Wojdyla D, Quintana R, et al. Applying the 2019 EULAR/ACR lupus criteria to patients from an established cohort: a Latin American perspective. RMD Open. 2020:e001097.
6. Ayano M, Horiuchi T. Complement as a biomarker for systemic lupus erythematosus. Biomolecules. 2023;13:367.
7. Gartshteyn Y, Mor A, Shimbo D, Khalili L, Kapoor T, Geraldino-Pardilla L, Alexander RV, Conklin J, Dervieux T, Askanase AD. Platelet bound complement Split product (PC4d) is a marker of platelet activation and arterial vascular events in systemic lupus erythematosus. Clin Immunol. 2021;228:108755.
8. Miyagawa T, Asano Y, de Mestier Y, Saigusa R, Taniguchi T, Yamashita T, et al. Serum H-Ficolin levels: clinical association with interstitial lung disease in patients with systemic sclerosis. J Dermatol. 2017;44:1168–71.
9. Khanna U, Galimberti F, Li Y, Fernandez AP. Dermatomyositis and malignancy: should all patients with dermatomyositis undergo malignancy screening? Ann Transl Med. 2021;9(5):432. https://doi.org/10.21037/atm-20-5215.
10. Aringer MSmolen JS. Mixed connective tissue disease: what is behind the curtain? Best Pract Res Clin Rheumatol. 2007;21:1037–49.
11. Weinstein A, Alexander RV, Zack DJ. A review of complement activation in SLE. Curr Rheumatol Rep. 2021;23:4–11.
12. Font J, Ramos-Casals M, Vilas AP, et al. Low values of creatine kinase in systemic lupus erythematosus. Clinical significance in 300 patients. Clin Exp Rheumatol. 2002;20:837–40.
13. Tiniakou E, Goldman D, Corse A, et al. Clinical and histopathological features of myositis in systemic lupus erythematosus. Lupus Sci Med. 2022;9:e000635. https://doi.org/10.1136/lupus-2021-000635.
14. Tselios K, Gladman DD, Su J, Urowitz MB. Antimalarials as a risk factor for elevated muscle enzymes in systemic lupus erythematosus. Lupus. 2016;25(5):532–5.
15. Silver EM, Ochoa W. Glucocorticoid-induced myopathy in a patient with systemic lupus erythematosus (SLE): a case report and review of the literature. Am J Case Rep. 2018;19:277–83.
16. Walker UA, Clements PJ, Allanore Y, Distler O, Oddis CV, Khanna D, Furst DE. Muscle involvement in systemic sclerosis: points to consider in clinical trials. Rheumatology. 2017;56(suppl_5):v38–44.
17. Siegert E, Uruha A, Goebel HH, et al. Systemic sclerosis-associated myositis features minimal inflammation and characteristic capillary pathology. Acta Neuropathol. 2021;141:917–27.
18. Yang SH, Chang C, Lian ZX. Polymyositis and dermatomyositis–challenges in diagnosis and management. J Trans Autoimmun. 2019;2:100018.
19. Kwan C, Milosevic S, Benham H, et al. A rare form of dermatomyositis associated with muscle weakness and normal creatine kinase level. BMJ Case Reports CP. 2020;13:e232260.
20. Lokesh S, Tony K, Suresh V, Malepati B. A rare case of mixed connective tissue disease (MCTD) with intricate features of lupus, polymyositis and rheumatoid arthritis presenting with severe myositis. J Clin Diagn Res. 2015;9(3):OD05.
21. Qudsiya Z, Waseem M. Dermatomyositis. [Updated 2022 Aug 8]. In: StatPearls [Internet]. Treasure Island (FL): StatPearls Publishing; 2023. Available from: https://www.ncbi.nlm.nih.gov/books/NBK558917/
22. Chanprapaph K, Tankunakorn J, Suchonwanit P, et al. Dermatologic manifestations, histologic features and disease progression among cutaneous lupus erythematosus subtypes: a prospective observational study in Asians. Dermatol Ther (Heidelb). 2021;11:131–47.
23. Makavos G, Varoudi M, Papangelopoulou K, Kapniari E, Plotas P, Ikonomidis I, Papadavid E. Echocardiography in autoimmune rheumatic diseases for diagnosis and prognosis of cardiovascular complications. Medicina (Kaunas). 2020;56(9):445.
24. Kamal DE, Fahmi DS, Abdelsalam NA, et al. Fragmented QRS complex, highly sensitive CRP, and fibrinogen in early detection of asymptomatic cardiac involvement in systemic lupus erythematosus. Egypt Rheumatol Rehabil. 2023;50:44.

25. Lee KI, Manuntag LJ, Kifayat A, Manuntag SE, Sperber K, Ash JY, Frishman WH, Wasserman A. Cardiovascular manifestations of systemic sclerosis: an overview of pathophysiology, screening modalities, and treatment options. Cardiol Rev. 2023;31(1):22–7.
26. Glynn P, Hale S, Hussain T, Freed BH. Cardiovascular imaging for systemic sclerosis monitoring and management. Front Cardiovasc Med. 2022;9:846213. https://doi.org/10.3389/fcvm.2022.846213.
27. Danieli MG, et al. Cardiac involvement in polymyositis and dermatomyositis. Autoimmun Rev. 2016; https://doi.org/10.1016/j.autrev.2016.01.015.
28. Choudhury S, Ramos M, Anjum H, et al. Shrinking lung syndrome: a rare manifestation of systemic lupus erythematosus. Cureus. 2020;12(5):e8216.
29. Cereser L, Passarotti E, De Pellegrin A, Patruno V, Di Poi E, Marchesini F, Zuiani C, Girometti R. Chest high-resolution computed tomography in patients with connective tissue disease: pulmonary conditions beyond "the usual suspects". Curr Probl Diagn Radiol. 2022;51(5):759–67.
30. Ruaro B, Santiago T, Hughes M, Lepri G, Poillucci G, Baratella E, Salton F, Confalonieri M. The updated role of ultrasound in assessing dermatological manifestations in systemic sclerosis. Open Access Rheumatol. 2021;13:79–91.
31. Hughes M, Moore T, Manning J, Dinsdale G, Herrick AL, Murray A. A pilot study using high-frequency ultrasound to measure digital ulcers: a possible outcome measure in systemic sclerosis clinical trials? Clin Exp Rheumatol. 2017;106(4):218–9.
32. Chatzinikolaou S-L, Quirk B, Murray C, Planche K. Radiological findings in gastrointestinal scleroderma. J Scleroderma Related Disorders. 2020;5(1):21–32. https://doi.org/10.1177/2397198319848550.
33. Jacques T, Sudoł-Szopińska I, Larkman N, O'Connor P, Cotten A. Musculoskeletal manifestations of non-RA connective tissue diseases: scleroderma, systemic lupus erythematosus, still's disease, Dermatomyositis/Polymyositis, Sjögren's syndrome, and mixed connective tissue disease. Semin Musculoskelet Radiol. 2018;22(2):166–79.
34. Lilleker JB, Vencovsky J, Wang G, et al. The EuroMyositis registry: an international collaborative tool to facilitate myositis research. Ann Rheum Dis. 2018;77(01):30–9.
35. Kang EH, Lee EB, Shin KC, Im CH, Chung DH, Han SK, et al. Interstitial lung disease in patients with polymyositis, dermatomyositis and amyopathic dermatomyositis. Rheumatology (Oxford). 2005;44(10):1282–6.
36. BellandoRandone S, Matucci-Cerinic M. Very early systemic sclerosis and pre-systemic sclerosis: definition, recognition, clinical relevance and future directions. Curr Rheumatol Rep. 2017;19(10):65.
37. Ciancio N, Pavone M, Torrisi SE, et al. Contribution of pulmonary function tests (PFTs) to the diagnosis and follow up of connective tissue diseases. Multidiscip Respir Med. 2019;14:17.
38. Thongpooswan S, Tushabe R, Song J, Kim P, Abrudescu A. Mixed connective tissue disease and papillary thyroid cancer: a case report. Am J Case Rep. 2015;16:517–9. https://doi.org/10.12659/AJCR.894176.
39. Cappelli LC, Shah AA. The relationships between cancer and autoimmune rheumatic diseases. Best Pract Res Clin Rheumatol. 2020; https://doi.org/10.1016/j.berh.2019.101472.

Part II

Approach Towards Specific Connective Tissue Diseases

5 Raynaud's Phenomenon

Ankan Gupta and Kriteeka Saini

Abstract

Raynaud's phenomenon is a relatively common vasospastic phenomenon in response to exposure to cold environment, emotional stress, or other physical or medication exposures. It is seen more commonly in women, during the second and third decades of life. It is a clinical diagnosis, characterized by classical triphasic color changes of the digits. It is important to differentiate primary Raynaud's disease from secondary Raynaud's phenomenon, as the latter is associated with complications such as digital ischemia and ulceration. All patients presenting with Raynaud's phenomenon should undergo complete evaluation including a nailfold capillaroscopy.

Keywords

Raynauds' phenomenon · Vasospasm · Nailfold capillaroscopy

5.1 Introduction

Raynaud's phenomenon (RP), named after the French physician Maurice Raynaud, is a disorder of microvasculature, presenting as an exaggerated vaso-occlusive disorder secondary to known triggers like cold, vibration, or emotional stress and manifests as sharply demarcated sequential color changes on acral skin. The term primary Raynaud's phenomenon (or Raynaud's disease) is used when secondary causes notably the connective tissue diseases and hematological malignancies have

A. Gupta (✉)
Department of Dermatology, Blacktown Dermatology, Sydney, NSW, Australia

K. Saini
Kavach Skin Clinic, Mhow, Madhya Pradesh, India

P. Agarwal et al. (eds.), *Dermatologist's Handbook of Autoimmune Connective Tissue Diseases*, https://doi.org/10.1007/978-981-95-0524-1_5

Table 5.1 Differences between primary and secondary Raynaud's phenomenon

	Primary RP	Secondary RP
Age of onset	Below 40 years	Above 40 years
Gender predilection	Female	Male
Distribution	Symmetric	Asymmetric
Attacks	Episodic, less painful	Frequent, more painful
Peripheral vascular disease	Absent	Present
Digital ulcers	Absent	Present
Digital pitting/scarring	Absent	Present
ANA	Negative	Positive
Inflammatory markers	Normal	Elevated
Nailfold capillaroscopy	Normal	Abnormal

been ruled out in an apparently healthy individual. It is a benign condition, rarely transient, but has a significant impact on patient's quality of life [1]. Table 5.1 elaborates the differences between primary and secondary Raynaud's phenomenon (Box 5.1).

Box 5.1: Risk Factors for Raynaud's Disease [1]

- Female gender.
- Positive family history in first-degree relative.
- Manual occupation.
- Smoking.
- Migraine.
- Estrogen replacement therapy.

5.2 Etiopathogenesis

There is a complex interplay of multiple factors such as vascular, intravascular, and neural abnormalities in the pathogenesis of RP. These factors may differ among those with primary versus secondary RP [2–4]. The interplay between various factors has been depicted in Fig. 5.1.

Secondary Raynaud's phenomenon, also referred to as Raynaud's syndrome, is seen in association with an underlying connective tissue disease like systemic lupus erythematosus, systemic sclerosis, Sjogren's syndrome, antiphospholipid syndrome, and drugs or occupational exposure. Table 5.2 gives a comprehensive list of the causes of secondary Raynaud's phenomenon. Various pathomechanisms have been suggested such as tumor invasion of sympathetic nerves, hyper-viscosity, hyper-coagulability, vasoactive tumor-secreted substances, generalized vasospasm, and spontaneous platelet aggregation [5].

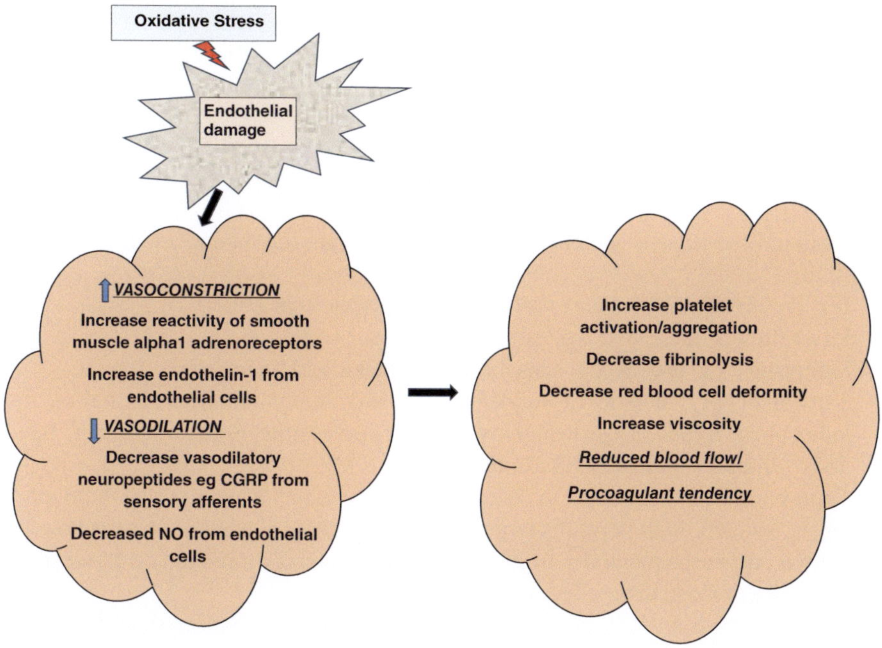

Fig. 5.1 Pathomechanisms involved in Raynaud's phenomenon

Table 5.2 Causes of secondary Raynaud's phenomenon [4]

Connective tissue disorders Scleroderma Systemic lupus erythematosus Sjogren syndrome Antiphospholipid syndrome	**Drugs** Ergot alkaloids Interferon alpha and beta Cyclosporine Nonselective beta blockers Clonidine Nicotine Chemotherapeutic agents: Bleomycin, erlotinib, cisplatin, vinblastine
Infections Parvovirus B19 Cytomegalovirus Hepatitis B Hepatitis C	**Occupation** Vibratory machinery: Jackhammers Exposure to polyvinyl chloride Cold injury from work Ammunition work
Obstructive vascular disease Thromboangiitis obliterans Microemboli Diabetic angiopathy Atherosclerosis Takayasu's arteritis Buerger's disease	**Hematologic causes** Cryoglobulinemia Cryofibrinogenemia Paraproteinemia Polycythemia
	Others Pheochromocytoma Carcinoid syndrome Hypothyroidism

Paraneoplastic Raynaud's Raynaud's as a paraneoplastic phenomenon has been reported in many carcinomas such as lung, breast, ovary, testes, skin, thyroid, sarcomas, and hematological malignancies.

5.3 Clinical Features [3, 4, 6]

- Raynaud's disease is seen mostly in females during the second and third decade of life.
- It is classically defined as a vaso-occlusive response in fingers.
- Sites: fingers, toes, nose tip, ears, and nipples.
- Symptoms: pin and needle sensation, numbness, and finger aches or pain.
- Typical history includes a single finger involvement initially, commonly the index or the middle finger which over time involves other digits of the same hand and eventually symmetrically in both hands.
- Thumb has been postulated to be a marker of secondary Raynaud's phenomenon.
- Onset: sudden, with painful sharply demarcated color change, better seen on the palmar surface sequentially from pale to cyanotic which turns red on rewarming, the entire episode lasting less than an hour [4].
- The classical triad of initial white (pallor from vasoconstriction), blue (cyanosis from sequestration of deoxygenated blood), and finally red (due to reperfusion and hyperemia) may not be seen in all patients.
- Primary RP is generally not associated with any visible sequelae; however repeated episode and chronic microangiopathy can lead to visible anatomical damage on fingers in the form of ulcers or gangrene.
- Secondary RP especially in systemic sclerosis is associated with severe episodes and visible sequelae such as digital ulcers.

5.4 Diagnosis

Raynaud's phenomenon remains a clinical diagnosis. In uncertain situation, standardized cold provocation test consists of exposing the hand to a temperature of 10 °C for 5 min and looking for color changes [7]. However, this is not recommended usually because of low reproducibility and a theoretical increase in microangiopathy with every demonstration (Fig. 5.2).

Nailfold capillaroscopy (NFC) is a useful bedside technique to differentiate primary and secondary Raynaud's and may facilitate very early diagnosis of a connective tissue disorder [8]. In patients with history and physical findings suggestive of a secondary cause, serological testing should be performed.

Basic laboratory investigations such as a full blood count, inflammatory markers, thyroid function, and ANA testing by indirect immunofluorescence should be tailored to the clinical findings [9]. Late age of onset, female gender, visible anatomical changes on finger tips, asymmetry in attacks in a long-standing disease, and changes of Raynaud's proximal to fingers warrant investigations for a secondary

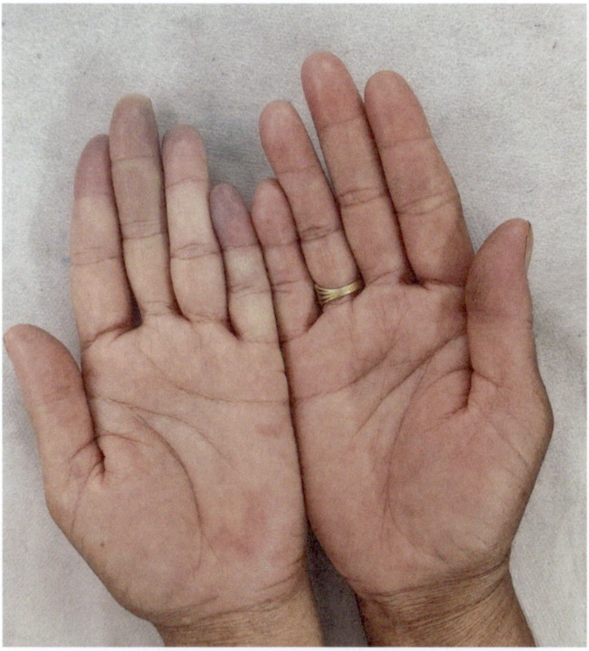

Fig. 5.2 Cold provocation test: right hand showing normal color without immersion; left hand showing color changes after immersion in cold water

causes [4, 6]. It is important to note that presence of Raynaud's with low positive antinuclear antibody result without any other clinical feature of a connective tissue disease is unlikely to be secondary Raynaud's and requires active non-intervention follow-up. Inflammatory markers, especially the erythrocyte sedimentation rate (ESR), are often serially checked [10].

5.5 Differential Diagnosis

Raynaud's phenomenon should be differentiated from other closely related acrosyndromes [11] (Box 5.2).

Box 5.2 Differential Diagnosis for Raynaud's Phenomenon

Condition	Differentiating feature
Physiological response to cold and stress	Symptoms mimic Raynaud's but **without** any color changes
Acrocyanosis	**Painless, persistent** bluish-red symmetrical discolorations of the hands, feet, and knees
Perniosis (chill blains)	Asymmetrical swelling, erythema, visible skin lesions in the form of **papules, blisters,** and cutaneous ulcers **Can last for days**. Accompanied with itching, burning or pain.

Raynaud's, acrocyanosis, and perniosis can coexist.

- Carpal tunnel syndrome is a commonly confused differential diagnosis; however it is an association of Raynaud's disease as well [12, 13].
- Occlusive vascular disease like small vessel thrombosis and vasculitis can mimic Raynaud's in early stages. Misidentification can have grave prognosis leading to tissue or digit loss as the tissue damage due to obliteration is often permanent.
- Peripheral neuropathy.

5.6 Nailfold Capillary Microscopy (NFC)

Nailfold capillaroscopy is an inexpensive, quick, and non-invasive technique that can help differentiate primary from secondary Raynaud's [4]. NFC analyzes the microvascular and morphologic changes in peripheral vessels such as changes in architecture, capillary size, capillary density, the presence of hemorrhage, and avascular areas [6]. NFC is done using a handheld or portable dermoscope (dermatoscope) and should be performed by a skilled clinician experienced in dermoscopy. Use of high-magnification nailfold video-capillaroscopy is restricted to research and is available in higher centers.

Secondary Raynaud's is suggested by the following findings in NFC[7]:

- Enlarged or distorted capillary loops.
- Capillary loss/dropouts.
- Loss of normal architecture of loops.

5.7 Conclusion

Raynaud's phenomenon is a common clinical syndrome with characteristic color changes in the digits as a result of vasospasm. Etiopathogenesis includes a complex interplay between vascular, intravascular, and neural factors. Common triggers include cold, vibration, or emotional stress. Primary Raynaud's phenomenon or Raynaud's disease should be differentiated from secondary Raynaud's which is often associated with underlying connective tissue diseases or due to certain medications. Raynaud's should also be differentiated from other acrosyndromes with characteristic color changes but with subtle differences in clinical presentation. All patients of Raynaud's should undergo comprehensive clinical assessment and investigations, including a nailfold capillaroscopy.

References

1. Garner R, Kumari R, Lanyon P, Doherty M, Zhang W. Prevalence, risk factors and associations of primary Raynaud's phenomenon: systematic review and meta-analysis of observational studies. BMJ Open. 2015;5(3) https://doi.org/10.1136/bmjopen-2014-006389.
2. Herrick AL. Pathogenesis of Raynaud's phenomenon. Rheumatology (Oxford). 2005;44(5):587–96. https://doi.org/10.1093/rheumatology/keh552.
3. Haque A, Hughes M. Raynaud's phenomenon. Clin Med (Lond). 2020;20(6):580–7. https://doi.org/10.7861/clinmed.2020-0754.
4. Temprano KK. A review of Raynaud's disease. Mo Med. 2016;113(2):123–6.
5. Madabhavi I, Revannasiddaiah S, Rastogi M, Gupta MK. Paraneoplastic Raynaud's phenomenon manifesting before the diagnosis of lung cancer. BMJ Case Rep. 2012;2012:bcr0320125985. https://doi.org/10.1136/bcr.03.2012.5985.
6. Musa R, Qurie A. Raynaud disease. In: *StatPearls*. StatPearls Publishing; 2022. http://www.ncbi.nlm.nih.gov/books/NBK499833/. Accessed 21 Feb 2023.
7. Naidu S, Baskerville PA, Goss DE, Roberts VC. Raynaud's phenomenon and cold stress testing: a new approach. Eur J Vasc Surg. 1994;8(5):567–73. https://doi.org/10.1016/s0950-821x(05)80592-4.
8. Lis-Święty A. Recent advances in the workup and management of Raynaud phenomenon. Pol Arch Intern Med. 2019;129(11):798–808. https://doi.org/10.20452/pamw.15008.
9. Pauling JD, Hughes M, Pope JE. Raynaud's phenomenon – an update on diagnosis, classification and management. Clin Rheumatol. 2019;38(12):3317–30. https://doi.org/10.1007/s10067-019-04745-5.
10. Maverakis E, Patel F, Kronenberg DG, et al. International consensus criteria for the diagnosis of Raynaud's phenomenon. J Autoimmun. 2014;48-49:60–5. https://doi.org/10.1016/j.jaut.2014.01.020.
11. Das S, Maiti A. Acrocyanosis: an overview. Indian J Dermatol. 2013;58(6):417–20. https://doi.org/10.4103/0019-5154.119946.
12. Cooke R, Lawson I, Gillibrand S, Cooke A. Carpal tunnel syndrome and Raynaud's phenomenon: a narrative review. Occup Med. 2022;72(3):170–6. https://doi.org/10.1093/occmed/kqab158.
13. Pal B, Keenan J, Misra HN, Moussa K, Morris J. Raynaud's phenomenon in idiopathic carpal tunnel syndrome. Scand J Rheumatol. 1996;25(3):143–5. https://doi.org/10.3109/03009749609080004.

Discoid Lupus Erythematous

6

Sudip Ghosh, Sharmistha Panja, and Partha Mukherjee

Abstract

Discoid lupus erythematosus (DLE) is the most common form of chronic cutaneous lupus erythematosus and can occur as an isolated entity or in association with systemic lupus erythematosus. The pathogenesis is multifactorial with a complex interplay between genetic predisposition and environmental triggers. Clinically, the lesions are erythematous, indurated plaques, having follicular plugging along with scarring and pigmentary changes. Photo-exposed areas are predominantly affected. It causes significant morbidity due to the scarring and pigmentary changes. Diagnosis relies mainly on clinical features, and early intervention is necessary to minimize long-term damage and improve quality of life.

Keywords

Discoid · Follicular plugging · Atrophy · Localized · Disseminated

6.1 Introduction

- Lupus erythematosus (LE) is a multisystem autoimmune connective tissue disorder that predominantly affects the skin and other internal organs.
- There are several types of cutaneous LE.

S. Ghosh (✉) · S. Panja
Department of Dermatology, Venereology, & Leprosy, R.G. Kar Medical College, Kolkata, West Bengal, India

P. Mukherjee
Department of Dermatology, Venereology, & Leprosy, College of Medicine & JNM Hospital, Kalyani, West Bengal, India

P. Agarwal et al. (eds.), *Dermatologist's Handbook of Autoimmune Connective Tissue Diseases*, https://doi.org/10.1007/978-981-95-0524-1_6

- Discoid lupus erythematosus (DLE) is a classic and the most common variant of cutaneous lupus erythematosus (CLE) that may occur independently or as a manifestation of systemic lupus erythematosus (SLE) in about 20% of cases.

6.2 Pathogenesis [1–4]

The pathogenesis of cutaneous DLE is multifactorial, and the interplay between genetic and environmental factors plays a vital role (Fig. 6.1). Among environmental factors, UVR is the most well-established trigger of both CLE and SLE, while the role of autoantibodies remains unclear in CLE. Patients with DLE have lower serum autoantibodies, such as antinuclear, anti-native DNA, anti-Sm, anti-Ro/SS-A, and anti-La/SS-B, when compared to patients with SLE and subacute cutaneous lupus erythematosus (SCLE). Several factors, outlined below, have recently been implicated in the pathogenesis of DLE.

- The increase of FasL (first apoptosis signal ligand) expression on inflammatory cells surrounding hair follicles plays a crucial role in the hair follicle damage that is specific to DLE. Apoptotic keratinocytes release pro-inflammatory molecules, contributing to tissue inflammation and autoimmunity, resulting in interface dermatitis in DLE.

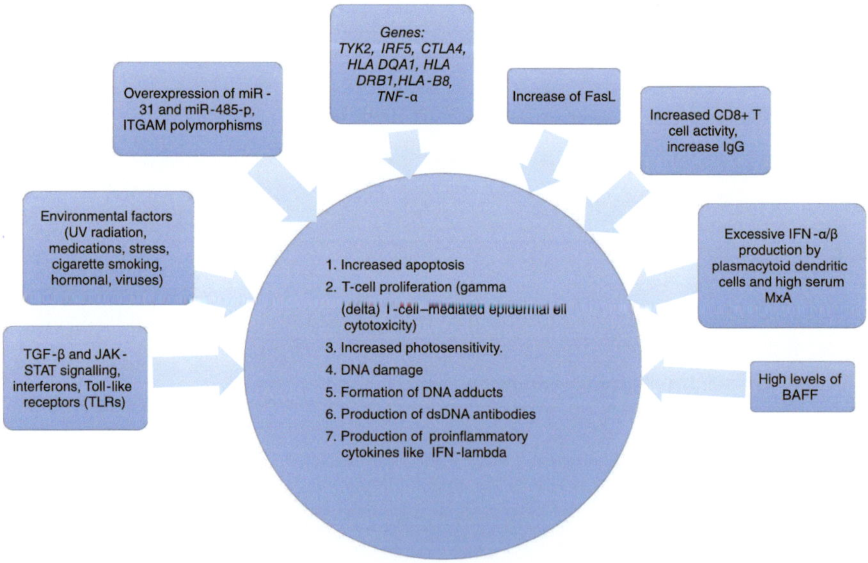

Fig. 6.1 Simplified pathogenesis of DLE (TGF-β, transforming growth factor-β; ITGAM, integrin alpha M; JAK-STAT, Janus kinase/signal transducer and activator of transcription; TYK2, tyrosine kinase 2; IRF5, interferon regulatory factor 5; CTLA-4, cytotoxic T-lymphocyte-associated protein 4; HLA, human leukocyte antigen)

- Excessive IFN-α/β production by plasmacytoid dendritic cells and high serum MxA (myxovirus resistance protein 1) levels are linked to inflammatory infiltration in LE lesions, especially in cutaneous LE-like disseminated DLE. Granzyme B levels are significantly elevated in CLE lesions at the dermo-epidermal junction and show a positive correlation with IFN-α expression. Dendritic cells (DCs) and natural killer (NK) cell-associated genes appear specific to inflamed skin in DLE patients. There is a correlation between plasmacytoid dendritic cell (pDC) increase and elevated inflammatory infiltrate in DLE skin damage. Increased CD8+ T cell activity is crucial in DLE initiation and may be responsible for scarring lesions. Nodular aggregates of B cell infiltrates in skin damage are common in DLE. Increased B cells have been found in patients with scarring lesions, indicating their role in scarring. High levels of BAFF (B-cell activating factor of TNF family) have been found in DLE skin damage, promoting B cells' survival.
- Frequently, IgM is the first to be recruited, and it attracts C3 and other immunoglobulins. While in cases of SLE, IgM alone or in combination with C3 is the most frequent form of immune complex formation, in DLE, IgG is responsible for the majority of immune complex deposits. IgG is the most commonly deposited immune complex in DLE, while IgM plays a much lesser role in skin damage.
- Previous studies have identified genes like human leukocyte antigens (HLA), interferon regulatory factor 5 (IRF5), Tumour Necrosis Factor alpha (TNF-α), and complement pathway genes as being linked to susceptibility to CLE. HLA variants are highly correlated with the disease progression of skin lupus. HLA-B8 positive can predict the progress from DLE to SLE, especially in female patients.

6.3 Types of DLE [5]

According to the modified Gilliam classification, DLE is a LE-specific lesion. It can be classified into several types (Table 6.1).

Table 6.1 Classification of DLE

(a) *Classic DLE*
(i) Localized DLE (80%)
(ii) Generalized DLE (20%)
(b) *Hypertrophic/verrucous DLE*
(c) *Lupus profundus*
(d) *Mucosal DLE*
(i) Oral DLE
(ii) Conjunctival DLE
(iii) Nasal DLE
(iv) Genital DLE
(e) *DLE-lichen planus overlap*

6.4 Clinical Features of DLE [6–8]

6.4.1 Symptoms

- Most patients are asymptomatic.
- Patients may experience mild pruritus, occasional pain, or burning within the lesions.
- Exacerbation is common with increased sun exposure, particularly in spring and summer.

6.4.2 Signs: Clinical Signs of DLE Are Tabulated in Table 6.2

Table 6.2 Clinical signs of DLE

Subtypes of DLE	Clinical features
Classic DLE	The lesions begin as infiltrated erythematous plaques, indurated on palpation, evolving with keratosis, mainly of follicular type, atrophy, and dyschromia, with hypochromia in the Centre with underlying telangiectasia and hyperchromia at the periphery. They are usually painful on palpation (Fig. 6.2) They can cause vitiligoid lesions, as well as scarring, often mutilating ones, especially when they affect the nose, ear pinnae, and eyelids. Lesions at different stages are often concomitant When located in hairy areas, such as the scalp, beard, eyelashes, and eyebrows, they tend to destroy the follicles, resulting in cicatricial alopecia (Fig. 6.3) Palmoplantar lesions are rare, usually very painful, and can ulcerate (Fig. 6.4) **Carpet tack sign/tin tack/cat tongue sign** By lifting the adherent scale from the lesion, follicle-sized keratotic spikes similar to carpet tacks can be seen to project from the undersurface of the scale **Schuster sign**—scarring lesions in the ear or Conchal bowl **Koebner phenomenon** can also occur in DLE
Hypertrophic DLE/ hyperkeratotic/ verrucous DLE	Exaggerated hyperkeratosis (Fig. 6.5) Extensor aspects of arms, upper back, and face are commonly affected
Mucosal DLE	Oral mucosa (commonest), conjunctival, nasal, genitalia (Fig. 6.6) 25% of CCLE
Overlap of DLE and lichen planus	Overlap of DLE and lichen planus can occur

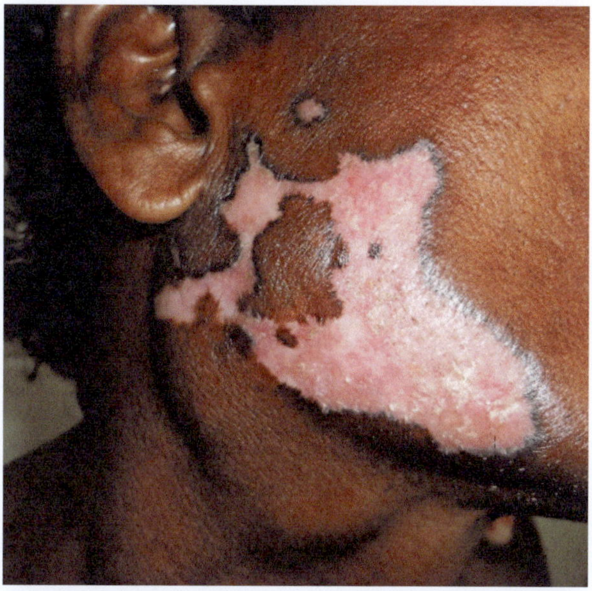

Fig. 6.2 Classic lesion of DLE

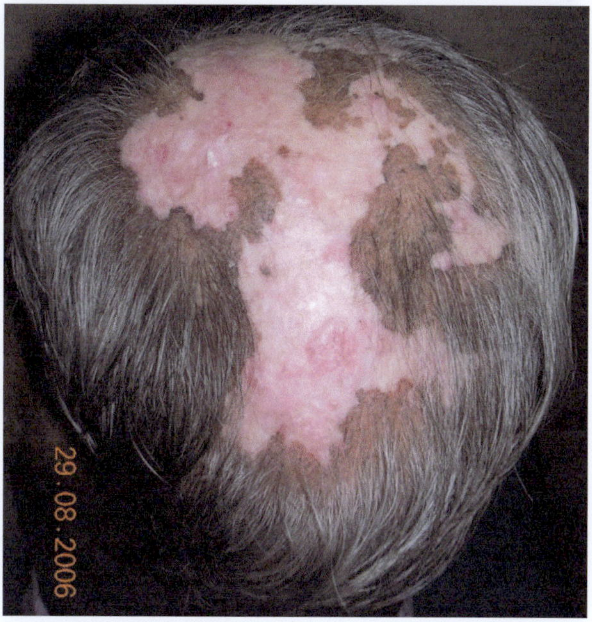

Fig. 6.3 Cicatrical alopecia over scalp due to DLE

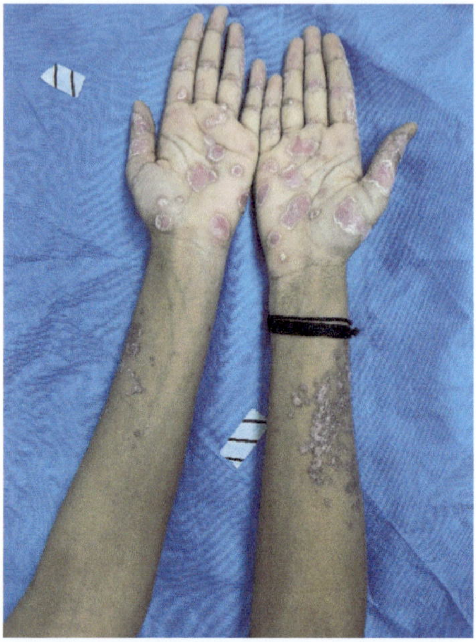

Fig. 6.4 Palmar lesions in DLE

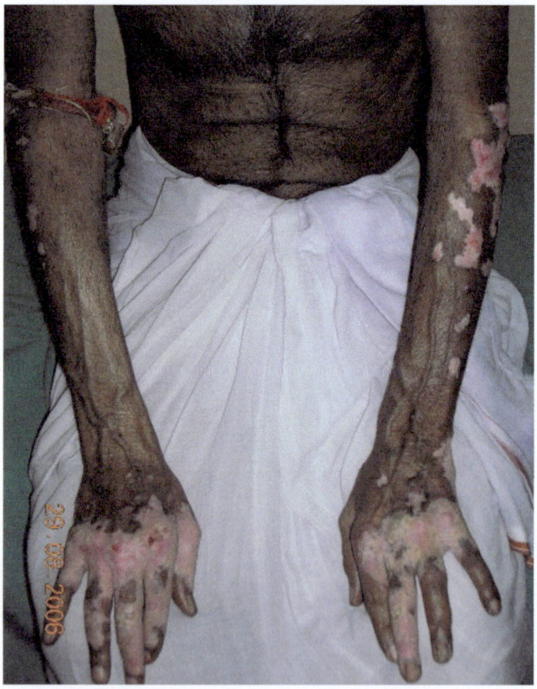

Fig. 6.5 Hypertrophic lesions of DLE over dorsa of hands

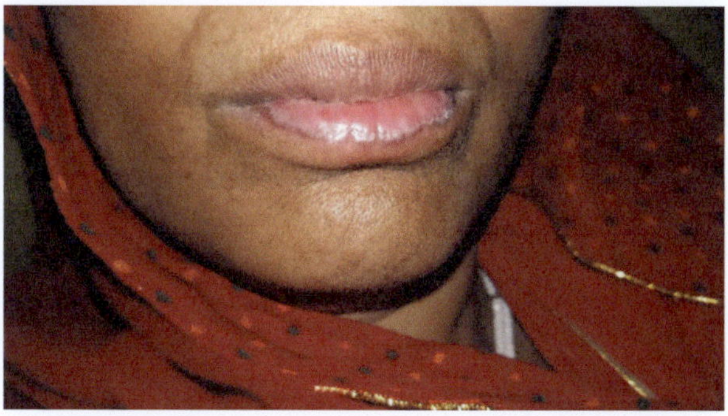

Fig. 6.6 DLE lesions over lower lips

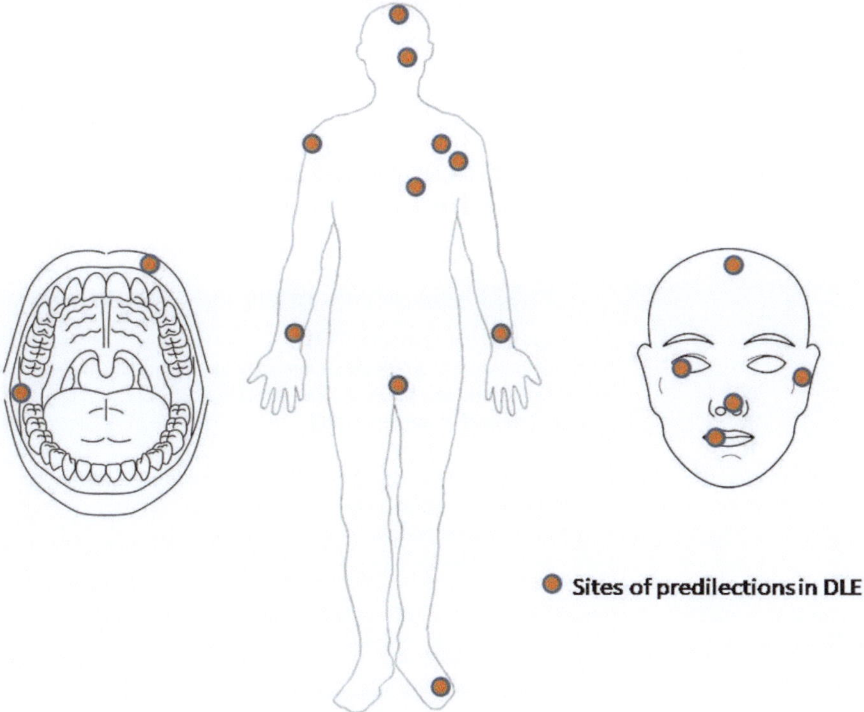

Fig. 6.7 Sites of predilection of DLE

6.4.3 Sites

- It is predominantly located on the head and neck, but in about 30% of cases, it can be disseminated and affect the trunk and limbs, with a preference for photo-exposed areas, such as the face, ear pinnae, V-neckline region, lateral cervical region, scalp, and dorsal region of the upper limbs (Fig. 6.7).

- Localized DLE is limited to sites above the neck. Generalized DLE refers to DLE occurring both above and below the neck.
- Occasionally, discoid lesions develop on mucosal surfaces, including the lips, nasal mucosa, conjunctivae, and genital mucosa.

6.5 Systemic Features [7]

- Patients who present with DLE may have associated arthralgias, but, over time, only approximately 10–20% of these patients ultimately meet the classification criteria for SLE.
- Approximately 5% of patients with localized and 20–28% with generalized DLE develop SLE.
- Patients with widespread involvement often have hematologic and serologic abnormalities.

6.6 Other Forms of Chronic Cutaneous Lupus Erythematous (CCLE) Are Summarized in Table 6.3

Table 6.3 Chronic cutaneous lupus erythematous other than DLE [9, 10]

Lupus tumidus	Also known as intermittent CCLE Erythematous, circular/annular, papules, and plaque with smooth surface; often urticarial-like presentation (Fig. 6.8) Tendency to heal without scarring Site: Face, neck, upper chest
Chilblain lupus	Red to dusky patches, papules to plaques, sometimes can present with ulceration, hyperkeratotic fissuring May present throughout the year Lesions exacerbated on exposure to cold Site: Acral areas, less frequently nose, ear, elbow, knuckles, knee
Lupus panniculitis (LEP)/profundus	Can present as separate or with SLE and DLE LEP co existing with DLE known as lupus profundus Tender to painful Subcutaneous indurated nodules/plaques May evolve into disfiguring, depressed areas Lesions of LE panniculitis typically have a distinctive distribution, occurring predominantly on the face, upper arms, upper trunk, breasts, buttocks, and thighs

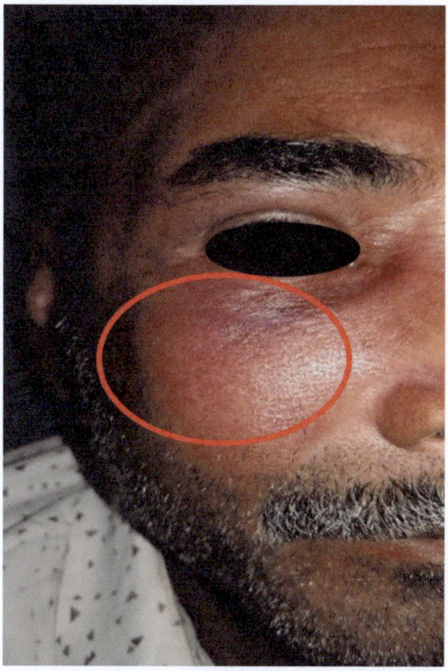

Fig. 6.8 Lupus tumidus

6.7 Classification Criteria: A 2020 Study Described the Validation of Classification Criteria for DLE (Table 6.4)

Table 6.4 Classification criteria for DLE [11]

Clinical feature	Points assigned[a]
Atrophic scarring	3
Location in the conchal bowl	2
Preference for head and neck	2
Dyspigmentation	1
Follicular hyperkeratosis/plugging	1
Erythematous to violaceous in colour	1

[a]A score of $\geq$5 points yields classification as DLE with 84.1% sensitivity and 75.9% specificity. A score of $\geq$7 points yield 73.9% sensitivity and 92.9% specificity

6.8 Methods for Severity Assessment [12]

- The Score of Activity and Damage in DLE **(SADDLE)** measures the severity of activity (erythema, scale, induration) and damage (scarring/atrophy and dyspigmentation) attributable to DLE.
- DQLI (Dermatology Life Quality Index).
- CLASI measures disease severity and responsiveness to therapy in cutaneous lupus erythematous.

The **CLASI-A score** (measures CLE activity) is generated by the clinician rating of erythema and scale/hypertrophy for each of 13 defined body areas—scalp ears, nose/malar area, rest of face, V-area neck (frontal), posterior neck and shoulders, chest, abdomen, back/buttocks, arms, hands, legs, and feet plus a rating for non-scarring alopecia. Scores represent the worst affected lesion within each area for each CLE-associated sign. In addition, the clinician seeks a yes/no response from the patient concerning hair loss in the past 30 days and current oral/nasal mucous membrane involvement followed by examination if the patient confirms involvement. The scores are calculated by simple addition based on the extent of each CLE-associated sign in specific anatomic areas.

The **CLASI-D (measures visible damage caused by CLE activity)** score is generated by the clinician rating of dyspigmentation and scarring/atrophy/damage due to resolved panniculitis for the same 13 body areas plus a score for scarring alopecia. The dyspigmentation score of 1 is doubled if the patient indicates the dyspigmentation usually lasts at least 12 months.

6.9 Differential Diagnoses [7]

Differential diagnoses of DLE are summarized in Fig. 6.9.

Clinicians often face a diagnostic challenge while differentiating malar rash or oral mucosal lesions due to acute LE or DLE. The clinical distinguishing features of acute LE and DLE with respect to malar rash and oral ulcer are discussed in Table 6.5.

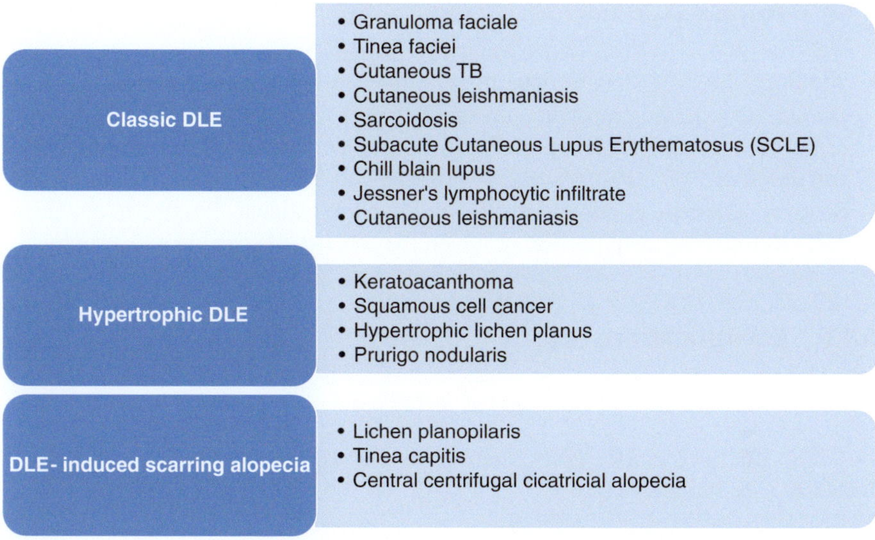

Fig. 6.9 Differential diagnosis of DLE

Table 6.5 Differentiating features of DLE and acute lupus erythematosus

Features	DLE	Acute lupus erythematosus
Malar rash	Induration present Relatively treatment-refractory	Usually no induration Relatively treatment-responsive
Oral mucosal ulcer	Usually painful. Well-demarcated White radiating hyperkeratotic striae Perilesional telangiectasia Honeycomb appearance Indurated The buccal mucosa is the most commonly involved site	Usually painless Less well-demarcated White radiating hyperkeratotic striae—Not seen Perilesional telangiectasia—Not present Honeycomb appearance Not seen Not indurated Palate is the most commonly involved site

6.10 Prognosis

- Although the prognosis of patients with discoid lupus erythematosus (DLE) is favourable regarding mortality, morbidity can be considerable.
- Many patients with DLE experience disfigurement from the scars or atrophy that can develop.
- Scarring alopecia is particularly distressing for patients. Prompt treatment of early lesions may help prevent or lessen the severity of scarring and atrophy.

6.11 Complications [7]

Complications of DLE are summarized in Table 6.6.

Table 6.6 Complications of DLE

Cutaneous	Cicatricial alopecia Dyspigmentation Squamous cell carcinoma
Extracutaneous	• *Haematological:* Pancytopenia, thromboembolism • *Rheumatological:* Arthritis, myositis • *Cardiorespiratory:* Hypertension, pleuropericarditis • *Renal:* Renal failure • *Ocular:* Optic neuritis • *Neuropsychiatric:* Depression, seizures • *GI:* Pancreatitis, mesenteric vasculitis • *Metabolic:* Vitamin D deficiency • *Iatrogenic:* Therapy-related adverse effects

6.12 Conclusion

Discoid lupus erythematosus is the commonest form of cutaneous LE. Depending on the extent, it can be localized or disseminated (DLE lesions involving below the neck also). Morphologically there are many variants, which include classic, hypertrophic or verrucous, mucosal, DLE-lichen planus overlap, lupus tumidus, lupus profundus, and chilblain lupus. It most commonly affects the sun-exposed areas with head and neck being the most common sites. The disease severity can be assessed through SADDLE (Score of Activity and Damage in DLE) and CLASI (Cutaneous LE Disease area and severity index) indices. Cosmetic disfigurement due to the scarring and pigmentation changes is one of the major causes of morbidity.

References

1. Vale ECSD, Garcia LC. Cutaneous lupus erythematosus: a review of etiopathogenic, clinical, diagnostic and therapeutic aspects. An Bras Dermatol. 2023;98(3):355–72. https://doi.org/10.1016/j.abd.2022.09.005.
2. Chen HW, Barber G, Chong BF. The genetic landscape of cutaneous lupus erythematosus. Front Med. 2022;9:916011. https://doi.org/10.3389/fmed.2022.916011.
3. Fijałkowska A, Kądziela M, Żebrowska A. The spectrum of cutaneous manifestations in lupus erythematosus: a comprehensive review. J Clin Med. 2024;13(8):2419. https://doi.org/10.3390/jcm13082419.
4. Millard LG, Rowell NR, Rajah SM. Histocompatibility antigens in discoid and systemic lupus erythematosus. Br J Dermatol. 1977;96(2):139–44. https://doi.org/10.1111/j.1365-2133.1977.tb12535.x.
5. Grönhagen CM, Nyberg F. Cutaneous lupus erythematosus: an update. Indian Dermatol Online J. 2014;5(1):7–13. https://doi.org/10.4103/2229-5178.126020.
6. Narang T, Sharma M, Gulati N, Kaur A. Extensive hypertrophic lupus erythematosus: atypical presentation. Indian J Dermatol. 2012;57(6):504. https://doi.org/10.4103/0019-5154.103085.
7. McDaniel B, Sukumaran S, Koritala T, et al. Discoid Lupus Erythematosus. [Updated 2023 Aug 28]. In: StatPearls [Internet]. Treasure Island (FL): StatPearls Publishing; 2025. Available from: https://www.ncbi.nlm.nih.gov/books/NBK493145/
8. Gopalan G, Gopinath SR, Kothandaramasamy R, Pandian S. A clinical and epidemiological study on discoid lupus erythematosus. Int J Res Dermatol. 2018;4:396–402.
9. Okon LG, Werth VP. Cutaneous lupus erythematosus: diagnosis and treatment. Best Pract Res Clin Rheumatol. 2013;27(3):391–404. https://doi.org/10.1016/j.berh.2013.07.008.
10. Rangel LK, Villa-Ruiz C, Lo K, Cobos G, Lo Sicco K, Vleugels RA, Femia AN. Clinical characteristics of lupus erythematosus panniculitis/Profundus: a retrospective review of 61 patients. JAMA Dermatol. 2020;156(11):1264–6. https://doi.org/10.1001/jamadermatol.2020.2797.
11. Elman SA, Joyce C, Braudis K, Chong BF, Fernandez AP, Furukawa F, Hasegawa M, Kim HJ, Li SJ, Lian CG, Szepietowski JC, Werth VP, Merola JF. Creation and validation of classification criteria for discoid lupus erythematosus. JAMA Dermatol. 2020;156(8):901–6. https://doi.org/10.1001/jamadermatol.2020.1698.
12. Guo LN, Perez-Chada LM, Borucki R, Nambudiri VE, Werth VP, Merola JF. Development of a working core outcome set for cutaneous lupus erythematosus: a practical approach to an urgent unmet need. Lupus Sci Med. 2021;8(1):e000529. https://doi.org/10.1136/lupus-2021-000529.

Systemic Lupus Erythematosus 7

Kabir Sardana, Siddharth Ghogate, and Ashish Jagati

Abstract

Systemic lupus erythematosus (SLE) is a chronic autoimmune disease characterized by multisystem involvement. It presents with a wide range of clinical manifestations, making diagnosis and management challenging. Advances in understanding the immunological basis of the disease have improved treatment outcomes, but challenges remain in achieving early diagnosis and personalized care. This review discusses the pathophysiology, clinical features, diagnostic criteria, management and prognosis with an emphasis on current therapeutic strategies.

Keywords

Bullous SLE · Drug-induced SLE · Neonatal LE · Rowell's syndrome · Systemic lupus erythematosus

K. Sardana (✉) · S. Ghogate
PGIMER, Dr. Ram Manohar Lohia Hospital, New Delhi, India

A. Jagati
Department of Skin & VD, Smt SCL General Hospital, Smt NHL Municipal Medical College, Ahmedabad, Gujarat, India

P. Agarwal et al. (eds.), *Dermatologist's Handbook of Autoimmune Connective Tissue Diseases*, https://doi.org/10.1007/978-981-95-0524-1_7

7.1 Introduction

Lupus erythematosus (LE) is an autoimmune connective tissue disorder that continues to baffle the medical community to this day. With its multimodal aetiology and myriad clinical presentations, lupus forms a challenging clinical entity even for the most astute clinicians. The four main types of lupus are neonatal lupus erythematosus (NLE); cutaneous lupus erythematosus (CLE); drug-induced lupus (DIL); and systemic lupus erythematosus (SLE) [1].

Skin is the second most common organ involved, and mucocutaneous involvement is often the first clinical manifestation of the disease; hence the role of dermatologist in the management is paramount.

Clinical features and management of discoid lupus erythematosus are discussed in Chaps. 6 and 14.

7.2 Aetiopathogenesis [2]

The aetiopathogenesis of LE is multifactorial and is briefly summarized in Fig. 7.1. Genetic factors (genes involved in IFN a and B cell stimulation), gender, hormonal factor, environmental factors, infection and drugs trigger the cascade of events in pathogenesis of lupus.

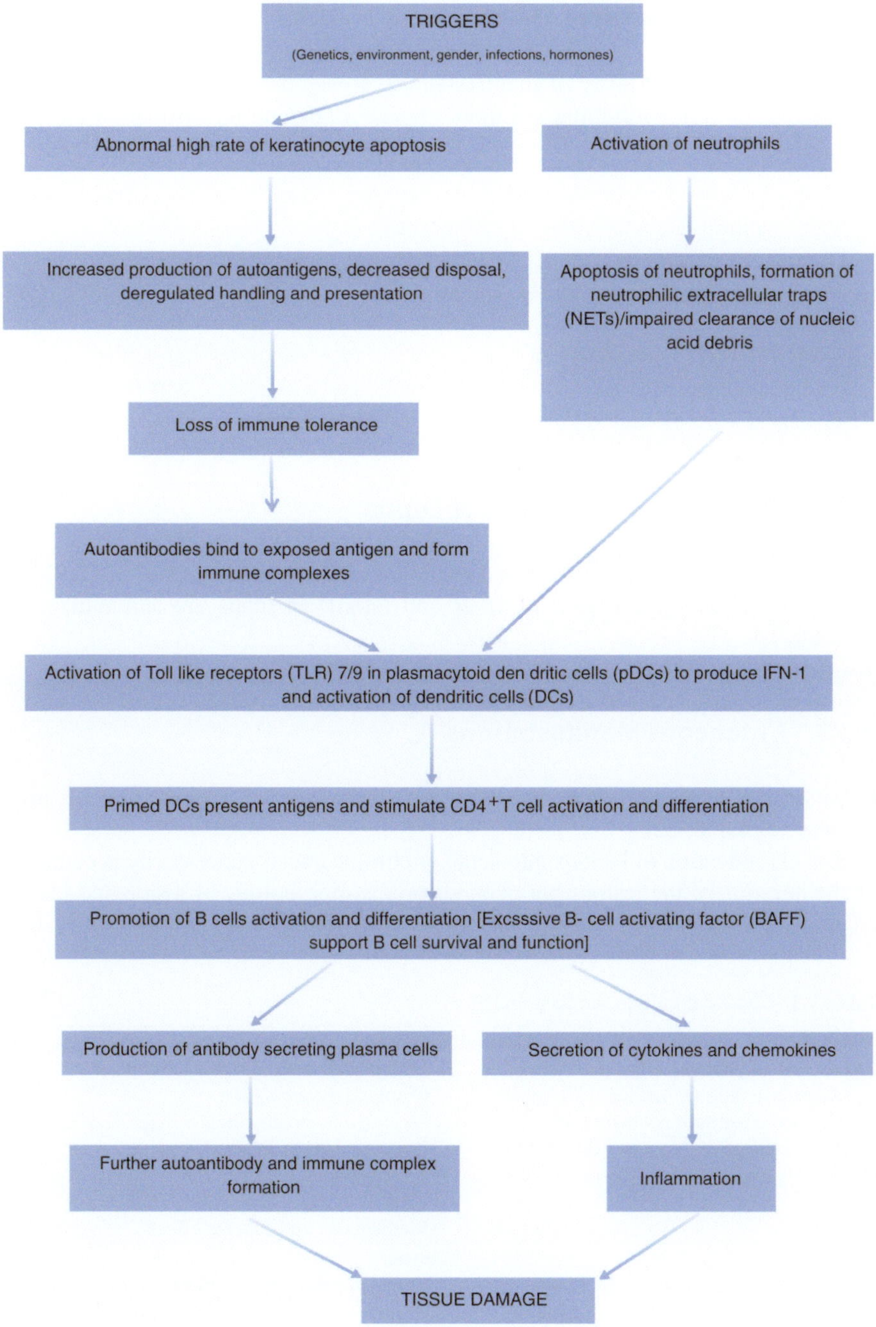

Fig. 7.1 Aetiopathogenesis of LE

7.3 Clinical Features [3–7]

As a result of its vast array of manifestations, it was thought that 'Lupus can do everything, but not everything is Lupus'; hence a law and its corollary were proposed (Box 7.1).

Box 7.1 Various Laws for Lupus Erythematosus
Greenwald's law—Everything that happens to a patient after being diagnosed as having systemic lupus erythematosus (SLE) is attributed to SLE, rightly or wrongly.

Sontheimer's corollary to Greenwald's law—Anything happening to a patient with positive ANA that is not immediately otherwise explicable will automatically be blamed on SLE.

7.3.1 General Manifestations of Lupus

- **Constitutional symptoms** are one of the most common features of SLE (90%).
- The prevalence and causes of fever and fatigue in lupus are summarized in Table 7.1.

7.3.2 Cutaneous Manifestations

- Cutaneous lupus was first classified by Gilliam into LE specific and LE non-specific (Table 7.2).
- The classification of lesions into acute or chronic doesn't necessarily account for the duration of the lesions but depends on the morphology of lesion and rate of progression.

Table 7.1 Causes of fatigue and fever in LE

Fatigue	**Causes**
67–90% of patients with lupus experience fatigue, making it the most common constitutional symptom [1] Being subjective, fatigue is difficult to quantify and must be assessed at each visit	Inflammation and disease activity Cytokine dysregulation Depression, anxiety (neuro-psychiatric LE) Systemic involvement Fibromyalgia Comorbidities Medications and adverse effects
Fever	**Causes**
Fever is reported to occur in 36–86% of patients with SLE, and 5% of patients with pyrexia of unknown origin eventually are diagnosed as SLE	Lupus disease activity: Most common cause of fever in SLE, though it should be labelled as a cause of fever only after excluding all other causes Infections: Increased susceptibility due to steroids and immunosuppressive agents

Table 7.2 Gilliam's classification of cutaneous LE

LE-specific lesions		
Acute cutaneous lupus erythematosus	Localized ACLE (malar rash) (Fig. 7.2)	Malar rash/butterfly rash Macular or maculopapular lesions which progress to confluent erythema present on the malar convexities, bridge of the nose with sparing of the nasolabial folds Unilateral involvement, forehead, periorbital area, chin and photo-exposed portion of neck may also be involved Generally heals without any scarring though post-inflammatory dyspigmentation may occur, particularly in darker skin types
	Generalized ACLE (Fig. 7.3)	More generalized form of the rash Exanthematous eruption involving the photo-exposed areas When the dorsa of fingers are involved, the erythema has a proclivity to spare the knuckles, aiding differentiation from Gottron's sign seen in dermatomyositis (DM) Perivascular nailfold erythema and telangiectasias may be present
	Toxic epidermal necrolysis like ACLE (Fig. 7.4)	Aptly christened as acute syndrome of apoptotic pan-epidermolysis (ASAP) syndrome Due to severe apoptosis leading to full thickness epidermal necrosis impersonating TEN Extensive mucosal ulceration may be present Predominant photo-exposed distribution of the lesions may assist differentiation from TEN Has an insidious onset and may have a prolonged course Absence of drug exposure differentiates it from classic TEN
SCLE	1. Annular SCLE. (1/third patients) (Fig. 7.5) 2. Papulosquamous/ psoriasiform SCLE. (2/third patients)	Strongly associated with anti-Ro/La antibodies Relative sparing of the midface with more peripheral involvement Lesions are more hyperkeratotic and less oedematous than ACLE Resolve with more pigmentary changes Maybe associated with RA, Sjögren's syndrome, drug exposure or occur as a paraneoplastic syndrome
Chronic cutaneous LE	Discussed in Chap. 6	

(continued)

Table 7.2 (continued)

Non-specific LE lesions	
Cutaneous vascular disease	1. Vasculitis (Fig. 7.6) Leukocytoclastic (palpable purpura/urticarial vasculitis) Polyarteritis nodosa like cutaneous lesions 2. Vasculopathy Degos disease like lesion Secondary atrophie blanche (livedoid vasculitis, livedo vasculitis)
	1. Periungual telangiectasias 2. Livedo reticularis 3. Thrombophlebitis 4. Raynaud's phenomenon 5. Erythromelalgia
Non-scarring alopecia	1. Lupus hair 2. Telogen effluvium 3. Alopecia areata
Sclerodactyly Rheumatoid nodules Calcinosis cutis LE non-specific bullous lesions Urticaria Papulonodular mucinosis Cutis laxa/anetoderma Leg ulcers Lichen planus Erythema multiforme Acanthosis nigricans	

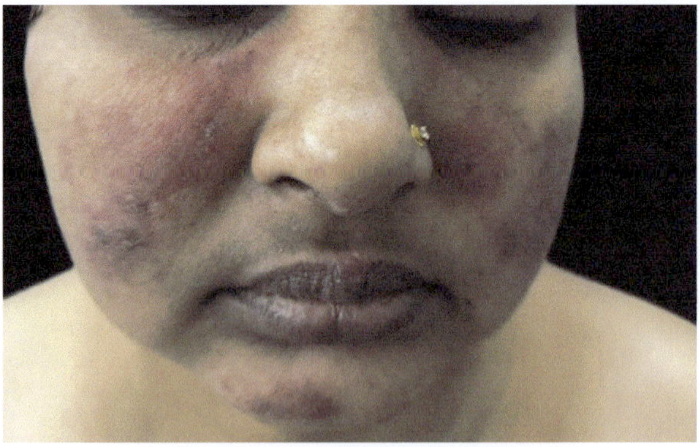

Fig. 7.2 Malar rash or butterfly rash

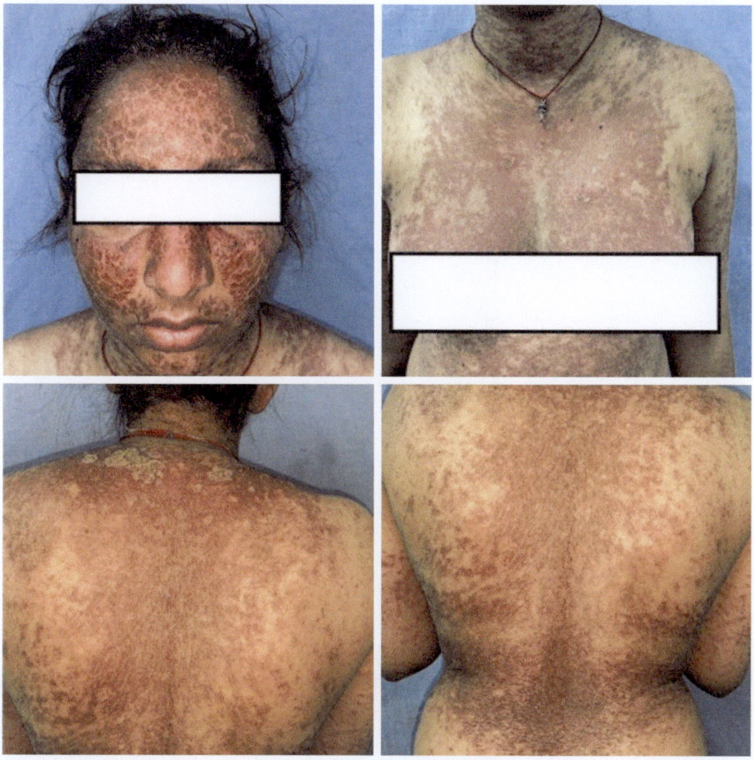

Fig. 7.3 Generalized ACLE

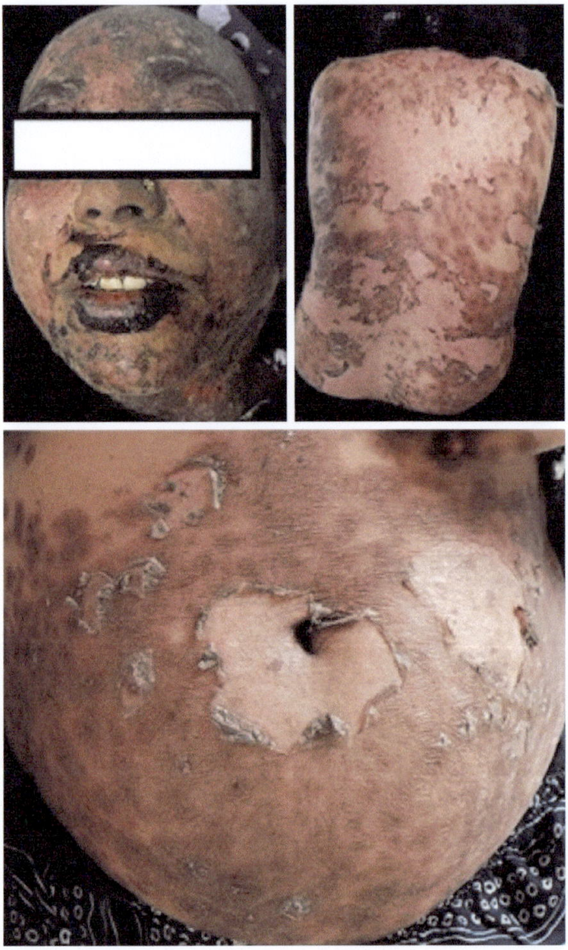

Fig. 7.4 Acute syndrome of apoptotic pan-epidermolysis (ASAP) syndrome or TEN-like ACLE

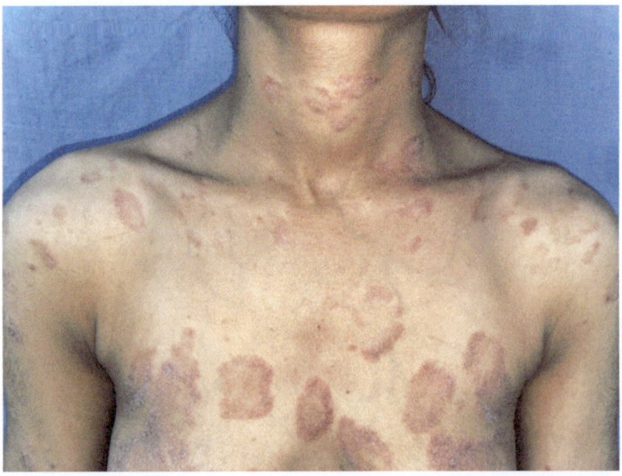

Fig. 7.5 Annular SCLE

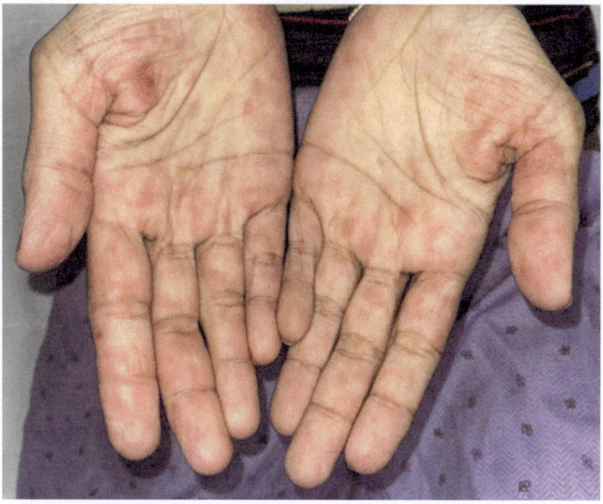

Fig. 7.6 Vasculitic lesions over palm

7.3.3 Hair Involvement in Lupus [8]

Lupus-associated alopecia can be both scarring (caused due to discoid lesions) and non-scarring which can be due to a variety of reasons (Fig. 7.7). Lupus hair are typically described as short lusterless brittle hair which impart a **'dishevelled appearance'** (Fig. 7.8). They are a marker of disease activity.

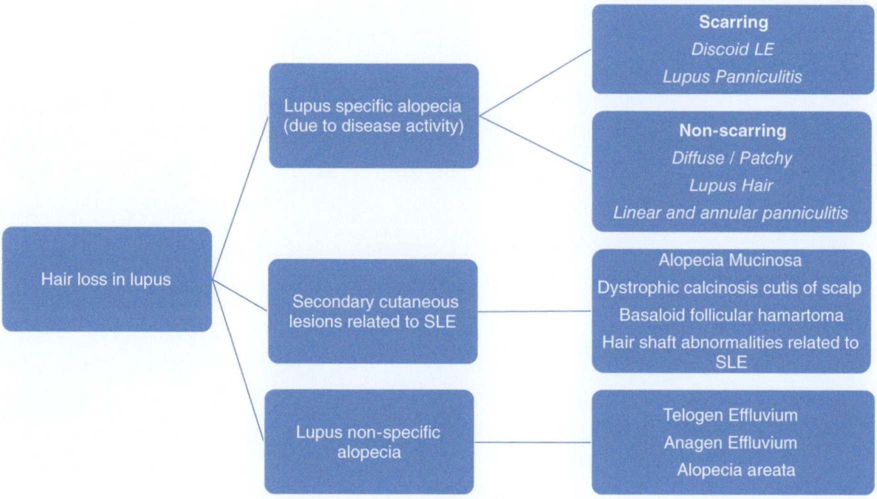

Fig. 7.7 Causes of hair loss in lupus

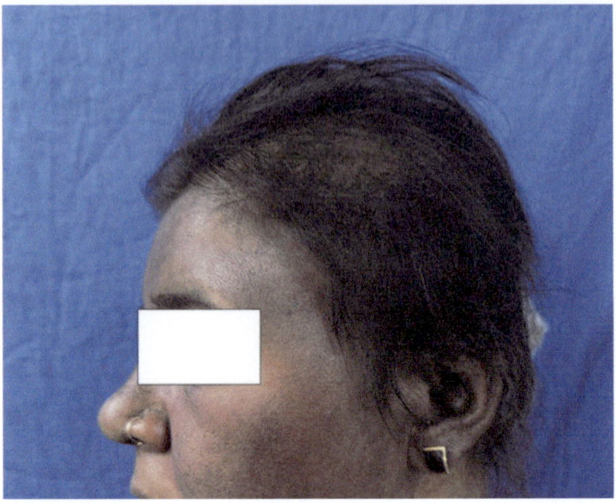

Fig. 7.8 Lupus hair

7.3.4 Mucosal Involvement [9]

Oral ulcers (Fig. 7.9) seen in SLE are usually painless (but may be painful) and more specifically present on the hard palate. The buccal mucosae may also be involved along with ulcers crossing the vermilion border of the lips. They may demonstrate perilesional erythema and keratotic hypertrophic striae extending outwards. The base is usually whitish and lacks slough.

Other manifestations of oral lupus include hyposalivation, gingival bleeding and petechiae.

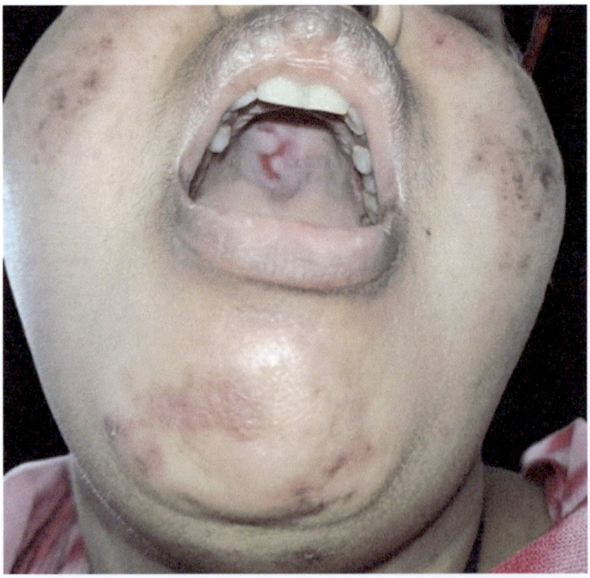

Fig. 7.9 Oral erosion

7.3.5 Musculoskeletal Involvement [10]

It is a very common manifestation of SLE and sometimes forms the earliest complain (Table 7.3).

Table 7.3 Musculoskeletal involvement in SLE

Arthritis and arthralgia	Can be one of the early presenting features Non-erosive, non-deforming, inflammatory symmetrical small joint predominant arthritis Early morning joint pain and stiffness in classic Dactylitis (sausage fingers or puffy fingers)
Jacound's arthropathy (JA)	Deforming arthropathy similar to rheumatoid arthritis occurring in nearly 35% of SLE patients [8] Joints of hands are involved with ulnar drift and metacarpophalangeal subluxation Reversibility of deformity differentiates it from true RA
Tenosynovitis	Reported in 10–13% of LE patients
Lupus myositis	Relatively rare Proximal upper limb and lower limb muscular weakness Could be due to Lupus itself (lupus myositis) Drug induced—Steroids, colchicine, HCQ, statins Fibromyalgia related Less elevation of muscle enzymes and fewer changes on biopsy differentiate it from inflammatory myositis
Osteonecrosis	Occurs in 5–12% of SLE cases Incidence decreasing to lesser use of prolonged corticosteroids AVN can occur due to: Systemic corticosteroids Raynaud's phenomenon causing ischaemia and necrosis Vasculitis Fat emboli Thrombosis due to APLA syndrome Groin pain worsened on weight bearing might indicate hip osteonecrosis, and the patient should be evaluated. A limping gait, with pain radiating to the thigh, could be a helpful pointer
Fibromyalgia	Prevalence of 15.8% in patients of lupus A syndrome with chronic fatigue and pain, sleep disturbances and functional symptoms

7.4 Other Systemic Manifestations [11–14]

Other system involvement has been briefly summarized in Table 7.4.

Renal Involvement in SLE [15]

- Renal involvement is more common than other systems in SLE.
- It can precede the diagnosis of SLE or occur during the course of treatment.
- Various reasons for kidney involvement in SLE are summarized in Table 7.5.

Table 7.4 Systemic involvement in SLE

Involvement	Clinical features
Central nervous system	
1. Aseptic meningitis	Photophobia, headache, neck stiffness, projectile vomiting which may be accompanied by fever Signs of meningism (Brudzinski and Kernig's sign) Important differential includes septic meningitis (increased risk due to immune dysfunction in SLE)
2. Cerebrovascular disease	Sudden onset neurological deficit: Motor weakness, loss of consciousness, falls, slurring of speech
3. Demyelinating syndrome	Lhermitte's sign may be positive
4. Headache	Red flag signs warranting investigations: Sudden onset headaches, onset after 50 years, positional headache, headache with neurological deficits, headache awaking patient from sleep, severe headache
5. Movement disorder	Chorea is the most common movement disorder in SLE Athetosis, hemiballismus, myoclonus, tremors, dystonia have all been described
6. Myelitis	Grey matter disease 1. Acute onset, with rapid deterioration in 6–8 h 2. Severe weakness at nadir, frequent bladder involvement, associated with active lupus 3. Poorer prognosis with irreversible paraplegia being possible White matter disease. 1. Subacute and indolent onset with slower progression 2. More hyperreflexia and spasticity
7. Myelopathy	Pain, paraesthesia, muscle weakness Band-like sensation around the abdomen is characteristic Sensory level is almost always present Bowel and bladder involvement is common
8. Seizures	Most frequently generalized tonic clonic seizures Status epilepticus
9. Mood disorders	Low mood/depression Anhedonia, disinterested Anxiety

(continued)

Table 7.4 (continued)

Involvement	Clinical features
10. Cognitive dysfunction	Memory difficulty termed as 'lupus fog' Personality change, impaired judgement, aphasia, apraxia
11. Psychosis	Delusions, hallucinations, confused talking May present de novo or with background SLE Steroid-induced psychosis forms a substantial differential Favourable prognosis with intensive immunosuppression
11. Reversible cerebral vasoconstriction syndrome	Sudden onset 'thunderclap headache' PRES (posterior reversible encephalopathy syndrome)
12. Vasculitis	Headache Stroke Seizures Psychiatric symptoms
Peripheral nervous system	
1. Axonal neuropathies: Polyneuropathy, cranial neuropathy, mononeuropathy, mononeuritis multiplex	Loss of sensations, paraesthesia, motor weakness and flaccid paralysis Cranial nerve involvement may cause blindness, ophthalmoplegia, ptosis, facial palsy, tinnitus, nystagmus, vertigo
2. Demyelinating neuropathies: Guillain-Barré syndrome like or sensory demyelinating polyneuropathy	Numbness and paraesthesia in the feet followed by ascending paralysis in AIDP
3. Autonomic disorder	Postural hypotension, headaches, constipation, erectile dysfunction, hypo−/anhidrosis
4. Myasthenia gravis	Fatiguability on repeated movement of muscles Muscle weakness, such as drooping eyelids more in the evenings Tendon reflexes are spared
Cardiac	
1. Pericarditis (with/without effusion)	Sharp precordial chest pain relived on bending forward Dyspnoea and palpitations may occur Pericardial friction rub may be present on auscultation
2. Myocarditis	Unexplained tachycardia, chest pain, palpitations or heart failure should arouse suspicion Unexplained ECG abnormalities may be present Clinical examination may show cardiomegaly and signs of heart failure
3. Valvular disease	Valvular regurgitation or stenosis may occur, with the mitral and aortic valves being affected more When a new murmur is auscultated, a transthoracic echo should be done to confirm the diagnosis Increased risk of incidence of stroke and embolism

(continued)

Table 7.4 (continued)

Involvement	Clinical features
4. Coronary artery disease	Angina and non-anginal chest pain Myocardial infarction may occur Coronary aneurysms may occur
Pulmonary	
1. Pleuritis and pleural effusion (PE)	Sharp, well-localized chest pain, which increases with inspiration, heralds a pleural effusion Auscultation might reveal pleural rubs PEs in SLE are frequently small, bilateral and exudative
2. Lupus pneumonitis	Fever, dyspnoea, cough, coughing, pleuritic chest pain and haemoptysis
3. Chronic interstitial lung disease	Exertional dyspnoea, non-productive cough and fatigue Basilar rales are heard on auscultation
4. Diffuse alveolar haemorrhage	Haemoptysis Acute onset pulmonary symptoms
5. Pulmonary embolism	
6. Pulmonary hypertension	Exertional dyspnoea and non-productive cough
7. Acute reversible hypoxemia syndrome	Described in patients experiencing SLE flare who are acutely ill Patients have hypoxemia and increased alveolar-arterial diffusion gradient in the absence of underlying chest radiograph and ventilation-perfusion lung scan abnormalities
8. Shrinking lung syndrome (due to diaphragmatic weakness)	Dyspnoea
Gastrointestinal	
1. Mesenteric vasculitis (MV)	Sudden onset severe abdominal pain due to thrombosis of larger vessels May also be insidious and occur intermittently over a period of weeks or months Gastrointestinal bleeding and perforation
2. Protein-losing enteropathy	Pedal oedema Ascites with transudative fluid
3. Peritonitis	May present as acute abdomen It is associated with disease activity
4. Lupus hepatitis	Usually, asymptomatic Fatigue, right upper quadrant discomfort, icterus
5. Lupus pancreatitis	Sudden onset severe abdominal pain radiating to back and relieved on forward bending Vomiting
6. Intestinal pseudo-obstruction	Abdominal pain Symptoms depend on the level of involvement, e.g. upper GI involvement causes nausea, vomiting and bloating Lower GI patients may have a delayed presentation with abdominal distention and constipation

(continued)

Table 7.4 (continued)

Involvement	Clinical features
Haematological	
1. Anaemia of chronic disease	Low haemoglobin Peripheral smear shows a normochromic, normocytic, hypoproliferative anaemia Low serum iron and low transferrin Normal to increased serum ferritin
2. Autoimmune haemolytic anaemia	Low haemoglobin Peripheral smear demonstrates spherocytosis Increased serum unconjugated bilirubin Raised lactate dehydrogenase (LDH) Increased reticulocyte count Reduced serum haptoglobin Direct coombs test is typically positive
3. Secondary immune thrombocytopenic purpura	Thrombocytopenia <50,000/mm^3 associated with active disease A subset of patients has mild thrombocytopenia, i.e. 250,000 to 150,000/mm^3, typically an isolated finding Chronic low-grade thrombocytopenia should raise suspicion of APLA Pentad of microangiopathic haemolytic anaemia, thrombocytopenia, CNS deficits, renal dysfunction and fever should raise suspicion of TTP
Thromboembolic	
1. APLA syndrome (Hughe's syndrome)	Cutaneous features: Livedo reticularis, livedo racemosa, leg ulcers, livedoid vasculopathy and atrophie blanche, gangrene of digits, nailfold infarcts, anetoderma, dermographism Deep venous thrombosis, pulmonary embolism, renal vein thrombosis, MI, stroke, sagittal sinus thrombosis, recurrent pregnancy loss Revised Sapporo criteria used for diagnosis
Lymphatic	
1. Reactive lymphadenopathy	Single or multiple, non-tender, mobile, discrete lymph nodes
2. Kikuchi-Fujimoto disease (histiocytic necrotising lymphadenitis)	Fever, night sweats and weight loss Tender cervical lymphadenopathy Resolves in 1 to 6 months without sequelae
Endocrine	
1. Hypothyroidism 2. **Hyperthyroidism**	Cold intolerance, dry xerotic yellowish skin, constipation, menorrhagia, weight gain, low mood **Heat intolerance, hyperhidrosis, weight loss with increased appetite, fine tremors, pretibial myxedema, acropachy**
Ocular	
1. Keratoconjunctivitis sicca and dry eye disease	Dry eyes, gritty foreign body sensation Conjunctival erythema, corneal erosions
2. SLE retinopathy	Sudden or gradual loss of vision
3. Episcleritis and scleritis	Redness of the eye, mild discomfort or soreness, tearing, light sensitivity
4. Uveitis and choroidal disease	Tender red eye with circumcorneal congestion

Table 7.5 Brief summary of renal involvement in SLE

Immune complex mediated	Non-immune complex mediated
Lupus nephritis (class I–V) Tubulointerstitial nephritis Renal vasculitis/vasculopathy Thrombotic microangiopathy With or without APLA	Glomerulosclerosis Hypertensive nephrosclerosis Amyloidosis Acute tubular necrosis (may be induced by rhabdomyolysis)
Nephritis due to associated disease Overlap syndrome ANCA-associated vasculitis Glomerulopathies due to sarcoidosis/IgA nephropathy	**Drug-induced renal involvement**

7.5 Variants of LE [8–10, 16–18]

- **Bullous SLE**
  - Subepidermal antibody-mediated blistering disorder.
  - Classified into type I (collagen VII antibodies present) and type II (antibodies to other DEJ proteins).
  - Distinct from blisters in ACLE, which are due to extensive epidermal necrosis.
  - Blister can occur on both photo-exposed and photoprotected sites.
- **Rowell's Syndrome**
  - Overlap of CLE with erythema nultiforme (EM) like target and targetoid lesions.
  - The diagnosis can be made with the help of the following criteria (Table 7.6).
- **Senear-Usher Syndrome (Pemphigus Erythematosus)**
  - Overlap between lupus erythematosus and pemphigus foliaceous.
  - Scaly plaques and rapidly healing blisters in seborrheic distribution reminiscent of pemphigus foliaceous with perinasal and malar erythema and discoid lesions.
  - Photosensitivity may be present.
  - ANA is positive in 30–80% of cases, and antibodies to Dsg 1 and Dsg 3 have also been described.

Table 7.6 Diagnostic criteria for Rowell's syndrome

Major criteria	Minor criteria
Presence of CCLE (DLE and/or chilblain) Presence of EM-like lesions (typical or atypical targets) At least one positivity among speckled ANA, anti-Ro/SSA and anti-La/SSB antibodies Negative DIF on lesional EM-like lesions	Absence of infectious or pharmacologic triggers Absence of typical EM location (acral and mucosal) Presence of at least one additional ARA criterion for diagnosis of SLE besides discoid rash and ANA and excluding photosensitivity, malar rash and oral ulcers
Diagnosis: Presence of all four major criteria and at least one minor criterion	

7.6 Diagnostic Criteria [19]

The 2019 EULAR/ACR classification criteria for SLE are the latest diagnostic criteria for SLE (Table 7.7).

Table 7.7 EULAR criteria for diagnosis of SLE

Entry criteria			
Anti-nuclear antibody (ANA) titre of ≥1:80 on Hep-2 cells or an equivalent positive test			
⇩			
If patient meets entry criteria, apply additive criteria			
Additive criteria			
Clinical criteria		**Immunological criteria**	
Clinical domains	**Weight**	**Immunology domains**	**Weight**
Constitutional 1. Fever	2	**Anti-phospholipid antibodies** 1. Anti-cardiolipin OR anti-β2GP1 OR lupus anticoagulant	 2
Haematological 1. Leukopeni 2. Thrombocytopenia. 3. Autoimmune haemolysis	3 4 4	**Complement proteins** 1. Low C3 OR C4 2. Low C3 AND C4	 3 4
Neuropsychiatric 1. Delirium 2. Psychosis 3. Seizure	2 3 5	**SLE-specific antibodies** 1. Anti-dsDNA antibody OR anti-smith antibody	 6
Mucocutaneous 1. Non-scarring alopecia 2. Oral ulcers 3. DL 4. SCLE 5. ACLE	2 2 4 4 6	1. Do not count a criterion if there is a more likely explanation than SLE 2. The occurrence of a criterion on at least one occasion is sufficient 3. SLE classification requires **at least one clinical criterion and ≥ 10 points** 4. Criteria need not co-occur **Only the highest weighted criterion is counted towards the total score within each domain**	
Serosal 1. Pleural or pericardial effusion 2. Acute pericarditis	5 6		
Musculoskeletal 1. Arthritis	6		
Renal 1. Proteinuria >0.5 g/24 h 2. Renal biopsy class II or V lupus nephritis 3. Renal biopsy class III or IV lupus nephritis	4 8 10		

7.7 Monitoring Disease Activity [20] (Table 7.8)

SLE Disease Activity Index (SLEDAI-2 K) is the most widely used index for monitoring the disease activity in SLE and is recommended by the European Alliance of Associations for Rheumatology (EULAR) also [13]. It scores various clinical and laboratory findings present in the past **10 days**.

Another index used in SLE is the Systemic Lupus International Collaborating Clinics/American College of Rheumatology (SLICC/ACR) Damage Index (SDI) developed in 1996. It is used to assess **permanent organ damage** in patients with **SLE** that has persisted for at least **6 months,** whether due to lupus itself or treatment side effects [21].

Table 7.8 SLE Disease Activity Index (SLEDAI-2 K)

Item	Definition	Score
Seizure	Recent onset, excludes metabolic, infectious or drug causes	8
Psychosis	Altered ability to function in normal activity due to severe disturbance in perception of reality	8
Organic brain syndrome	Altered mental function with impaired orientation, memory or other intellectual function. Exclude metabolic, infectious or drug issues	8
Visual disturbance	Retinal changes due to lupus	8
Cranial nerve disorder	New onset of sensory or motor neuropathy involving cranial nerves	8
Lupus headache	Severe, persistent headache due to lupus nonresponsive to narcotic analgesia	8
Cerebrovascular accident (CVA)	New onset of CVA. Exclude atherosclerosis	8
Vasculitis	Ulceration, gangrene, tender finger nodules, periungual infarction, splinter haemorrhages or biopsy-confirmed vasculitis	8
Arthritis	Joint inflammation in ≥2 joints	4
Myositis	Proximal muscle weakness with elevated muscle enzymes or electromyogram changes or biopsy-confirmed myositis	4
Urinary casts	Presence of red cell, granular, or mixed casts	4
Haematuria	≥5 RBCs per high power field (if not due to other causes)	4
Proteinuria	≥0.5 g/24 hours (new/worsening)	4
Pyuria	≥5 WBCs per high power field (exclude infection)	4
Rash	New or active lupus rash	2
Alopecia	Abnormal patchy or diffuse hair loss	2
Mucosal ulcers	Oral or nasal ulcers	2
Pleurisy	Pleuritic pain with pleural rub or effusion or pleural thickening	2
Pericarditis	Pericardial pain with at least one of the following: Rub, effusion or electrocardiogram or echocardiogram confirmation	2
Low complement (C3, C4)	Decreased CH50, C3 or C4 levels	2
Increased DNA binding	Increased anti-dsDNA by Farr assay	2
Fever	>38 °C (lupus-related)	1
Thrombocytopenia	Platelets <100,000/mm^3 (exclude drug causes)	1
Leukopenia	WBC <3000/mm^3 (exclude drug causes)	1

Scoring interpretation

0: No activity—No active lupus disease

1–5: Mild disease activity—Minimal lupus activity, may not require treatment changes

6–10: Moderate disease activity—Increased lupus activity, treatment adjustment may be needed

11–19: High disease activity—Significant disease activity, requires stronger therapy

≥20: Very high disease activity—Severe lupus flare, often requiring aggressive treatment.

7.8 Difference Between Systemic Lupus Erythematosus (SLE), Neonatal Lupus Erythematosus (NLE) and Drug-Induced Lupus Erythematosus (DIL) Are Summarized in Table 7.9

Table 7.9 Difference between systemic lupus erythematosus, neonatal lupus erythematosus and drug-induced lupus erythematosus [22–26]

	Systemic lupus erythematosus	Neonatal lupus erythematosus	Drug-induced lupus erythematosus
Pathogenesis	Multifactorial including genetic, environmental, hormonal factor (discussed above in detail)	Neonates with mother positive for HLA B8 and DR3- **predisposed to** NLE-positive for DRB-1*13 and Cw*06 **protected from NLE** Maternal IgG autoantibody against SSA/Ro, SSB/La and U1RNP passively transfer from placenta via FcRn receptor; binds to target organs causing tissue injury Defective phagocytosis of apoptotic cardiomyocyte and release of cytokines (TNF-α and TGF-β) results in inflammatory process causing conduction defect and fibrotic changes One of the suggested mechanism for cutaneous injury is overexpression of Ro antigen on keratinocyte The extent of tissue injury in neonate is directly proportionate to the titre of autoantibodies in the mother and all the neonates exposed to these autoantibodies will not develop NLE	Interplay between **genetic predisposition** (slow acetylation, association with HLA DR4, DR0301, Complement C4 null allele) **Drug biotransformation** (direct cytotoxicity) **Epigenetic dysregulation** (autoreactive T cells or B cell)

Mucocutaneous and systemic manifestation	**Cutaneous** Malar rash Photosensitivity Oral ulcer Alopecia **Systemic** Multisystem disease including Nephritis Neuropsychiatric (NPSLE) Musculoskeletal Cardiac	Cutaneous manifestations are common followed by cardiac and hepatic **Cutaneous** SCLE like erythematous annular/polycyclic lesion with/without scale mainly over face (periorbital and malar area –'owl's eye' or 'racoon' sign), scalp, neck. **Cardiac** Conduction abnormalities Myocarditis or cardiomyopathy **Hepatic** Elevated liver enzymes Conjugated hyperbilirubinemia **Haematological abnormality** Thrombocytopenia Rarely, neurological, haematological and spleen involvement	**More common** constitutional symptom, Myalgia arthritis, Serositis **Rare** Malar rash, nephritis and NPSLE **SCLE-DIL** with hydrochlorothiazide, diltiazem, verapamil, oxprenolol, terbinafine, antihistamines, immunomodulators, proton pump inhibitors, nonsteroidal anti-inflammatory drugs **SLE like DIL** hydralazine, procainamide, isoniazid, minocycline

(continued)

Table 7.9 (continued)

		Systemic lupus erythematosus	Neonatal lupus erythematosus	Drug-induced lupus erythematosus
Immunological workup	ANA	Positive in majority	Same as idiopathic SLE in mother	Positive in majority
	ANTI-ENA	Positive in different clinical subsets	**52/60-kD Ro/SSA and 48-kD La/SSB—**Associated with heart block **50-kD La/SSB** associated with cutaneous manifestation **Anti-U1RNP—**Atypical cutaneous lesion without cardiac or systemic abnormality and associated with thrombocytopenia	Rarely SSA and SSB
	ANTI-ds DNA	Positive	Same as idiopathic SLE in mother	Rarely positive (with anti TNF)
	ANTI HISTONE	Positive	Same as idiopathic SLE in mother	More frequently positive than idiopathic LE
	COMPLEMENT LEVEL	Low	Same as idiopathic SLE in mother	Rarely low
	pANCA, ANTI-MPO	Negative	Same as idiopathic SLE in mother	Seen with minocycline associated LE
Prognosis		Can be severe	Depends on the organs involved Cutaneous, haematological and hepatic disease is often transient with good outcome Some children with heart block may be well until adolescence at which point they develop syncopal episodes and require a pacemaker Children requiring pacemakers are at risk of cardiomyopathy later in life	Milder form

Treatment	Management according to recommendation	**Cardiac manifestations—**Regular monitoring by paediatric cardiologist Permanent pacemaker insertion when indicated **Cutaneous features—**Resolve spontaneously as maternal antibodies clear from circulation, i.e. 6–8 months Photoprotection Emollients for scaly lesions Topical corticosteroids may be considered for inflammatory lesions **Hepatobiliary disease** monitor Disappear spontaneously by 6–8 months Rarely, systemic corticosteroids, intravenous immunoglobulin may be considered but evidence of efficacy is lacking **Neurological abnormalities** Routine development assessment and serial head circumference measurement to monitor for hydrocephalus	Discontinuation of the causative drug **Mild cases**—NSAIDs or low doses of corticosteroid **Severe cases**—High dose of steroid or immunosuppressive **Topical steroid** for cutaneous lesions
Evolution	Chronic course	NLE with cutaneous involvement only—Excellent prognosis With cardiac involvement—20–30% mortality in the neonatal period With hepatic involvement—Transient liver disease but liver failure in severe involvement	Respond well both clinically and immunologically

7.9 Conclusion

Knowledge of extra-cutaneous manifestations in a patient suspected of having lupus erythematous will help in appropriately working up and referring the patient to allied super-speciality. For the rheumatologists, it is difficult to understand the rash and the differential diagnosis of other dermatoses mimicking malar and discoid rash. This chapter would help the physicians practicing both specialities in better understanding of clinical presentation of the lupus erythematosus.

References

1. Maidhof W, Hilas O. Lupus: an overview of the disease and management options. Pharmacy Ther. 2012;37:240–9.
2. Crow MK. Pathogenesis of systemic lupus erythematosus: risks, mechanisms and therapeutic targets. Ann Rheum Dis. 2023;82:999–1014.
3. Sontheimer RD. Greenwald's law of lupus: the Sontheimer amendment. J Rheumatol. 1993;20:1258–9.
4. Cleanthous S, Tyagi M, Isenberg D, Newman S. What do we know about self-reported fatigue in systemic lupus erythematosus? Lupus. 2012;21:465–76.
5. Timlin H, Syed A, Haque U, Adler B, Law G, Machireddy K, Manno R. Fevers in adult lupus patients. Cureus. 2018;10(1)
6. Ting W, Stone MS, Racila D, Scofield RH, Sontheimer RD. Toxic epidermal necrolysis-like acute cutaneous lupus erythematosus and the spectrum of the acute syndrome of apoptotic pan-epidermolysis (ASAP): a case report, concept review and proposal for new classification of lupus erythematosus vesiculobullous skin lesions. Lupus. 2004;13:941–50.
7. Sontheimer RD. Subacute cutaneous lupus erythematosus: 25-year evolution of a prototypic subset (subphenotype) of lupus erythematosus defined by characteristic cutaneous, pathological, immunological, and genetic findings. Autoimmun Rev. 2005;4:253–63.
8. Concha JSS, Werth VP. Alopecias in lupus erythematosus. Lupus Sci Med. 2018;5:e000291.
9. Burge SM, Frith PA, Juniper RP, Wojnarowska F. Mucosal involvement in systemic and chronic cutaneous lupus erythematosus. Br J Dermatol. 1989;121:727–41.
10. Ceccarelli F, Massaro L, Perricone C, Pendolino M, Cipriano E, Truglia S, et al. Jaccoud's arthropathy in systemic lupus erythematosus: clinical, laboratory and ultrasonographic features. Clin Exp Rheumatol. 2017;35:674–7.
11. Costa ACM, Dpf N, Júlio PR, Marchi-Silva R, De Aquino BM, De Oliveira AS, et al. Neuropsychiatric manifestations in systemic lupus erythematosus and Sjogren's disease. Autoimmun Rev. 2025;24:103756.
12. Tincani A, Rebaioli CB, Taglietti M, Shoenfeld Y. Heart Involvement in systemic lupus erythematosus, anti-phospholipid syndrome and neonatal lupus. Rheumatology. 2006;45:8–13.
13. Kamen DL, Strange C. Pulmonary manifestations of systemic lupus erythematosus. Clin Chest Med. 2010;31:479–88.
14. Cojocaru M, Cojocaru IM, Silosi I, Vrabie CD. Manifestations of systemic lupus erythematosus. Maedica (Bucur). 2011;6:330–6.
15. Pereira Rêgo Muniz M, et al. Renal involvement in systemic lupus erythematosus: additional histopathological lesions. Arch Med Sci. 2023;19:1398–409.
16. Yell JA, Wojnarowska F. Bullous skin disease in lupus erythematosus. Lupus. 1997;6:112–21.
17. Torchia D, Romanelli P, Kerdel FA. Erythema multiforme and Stevens-Johnson syndrome/ toxic epidermal necrolysis associated with lupus erythematosus. J Am Acad Dermatol. 2012;67:417–21.

18. Pérez-Pérez ME, Avalos-Díaz E, Herrera-Esparza R. Autoantibodies in Senear-usher syndrome: cross-reactivity or multiple autoimmunity? Autoimmune Dis. 2012;2012:296214.
19. Aringer M, Costenbader K, Daikh D, Brinks R, Mosca M, Ramsey-Goldman R, Smolen JS, Wofsy D, Boumpas DT, Kamen DL, Jayne D, Cervera R, Costedoat-Chalumeau N, Diamond B, Gladman DD, Hahn B, Hiepe F, Jacobsen S, Khanna D, Lerstrøm K, Massarotti E, McCune J, Ruiz-Irastorza G, Sanchez-Guerrero J, Schneider M, Urowitz M, Bertsias G, Hoyer BF, Leuchten N, Tani C, Tedeschi SK, Touma Z, Schmajuk G, Anic B, Assan F, Chan TM, Clarke AE, Crow MK, Czirják L, Doria A, Graninger W, Halda-Kiss B, Hasni S, Izmirly PM, Jung M, Kumánovics G, Mariette X, Padjen I, Pego-Reigosa JM, Romero-Diaz J, Rúa-Figueroa Fernández Í, Seror R, Stummvoll GH, Tanaka Y, Tektonidou MG, Vasconcelos C, Vital EM, Wallace DJ, Yavuz S, Meroni PL, Fritzler MJ, Naden R, Dörner T, Johnson SR. 2019 European league against rheumatism/American College of Rheumatology Classification Criteria for systemic lupus erythematosus. Arthritis Rheumatol. 2019;71:1400–12.
20. Gladman DD, Ibañez D, Urowitz MB. Systemic lupus erythematosus disease activity index 2000. J Rheumatol. 2002;29:288–91.
21. Ghazali WSW, Daud SMM, Mohammad N, Wong KK. Slicc damage index score in systemic lupus erythematosus patients and its associated factors. Medicine (Baltimore). 2018;97:e12787.
22. Lun Hon K, Leung AK. Neonatal lupus erythematosus. Autoimmune Dis. 2012;2012(1):301274.
23. He Y, Sawalha AH. Drug-induced lupus erythematosus: an update on drugs and mechanisms. Curr Opin Rheumatol. 2018;30:490–7.
24. Bilewicz-Stebel M, Miziołek B, Bergler-Czop B, Stańkowska A. Drug-induced subacute cutaneous lupus erythematosus caused by a topical Beta blocker – Timolol. Acta Dermatovenerol Croat. 2018;26:44–7.
25. Brockow KN, Khan DA, Banerji A. Drug allergy: definitions and phenotypes. In: Drug allergy testing; 2018. p. 19–26.
26. Miliaresis C, Izmirly PM, Buyon JP, Phoon CK, Friedman D. Neonatal lupus: pathogenesis and clinical approaches. In: Dubois' lupus erythematosus and related syndromes; 2019. p. 486–98.

Systemic Sclerosis 8

Pooja Agarwal

Abstract

Systemic sclerosis (SSc) is a complex autoimmune connective tissue disorder characterized by fibrosis, vascular abnormalities and immune dysregulation. It affects multiple organ systems and presents with a wide spectrum of clinical manifestations. Cutaneous involvement progresses through ill-defined stages, with Raynaud's phenomenon often being the earliest sign. Facial changes, digital ulcers, sclerodactyly, pigmentary alterations, nail abnormalities and calcinosis are key dermatologic features. Systemic manifestations include gastrointestinal involvement, pulmonary complications such as interstitial lung disease and pulmonary hypertension, cardiac abnormalities, renal crisis and musculoskeletal features.

Given its high morbidity and mortality, early diagnosis is critical, and dermatologists play a pivotal role in identifying initial cutaneous signs. Advancements in understanding the pathogenesis and risk factors have improved management strategies, but SSc remains a challenging condition with significant clinical variability.

Keywords

Prescleroderma · Systemic sclerosis · Skin thickening · Systemic involvement · VEDOSS

P. Agarwal (✉)
Department of Skin & VD, SVPIMSR, Smt NHL Municipal Medical College, Ahmedabad, Gujarat, India

P. Agarwal et al. (eds.), *Dermatologist's Handbook of Autoimmune Connective Tissue Diseases*, https://doi.org/10.1007/978-981-95-0524-1_8

Synonyms
Scleroderma; Progressive systemic sclerosis.

8.1 Introduction

Systemic sclerosis (SSc) is an autoimmune connective tissue disorder involving multiple systems. The synonym *scleroderma* does not completely justify the disease as it can be best understood as an umbrella term for any disease which has sclerosis of the skin (including morphea, etc.) and is best avoided.

- *SSc sine scleroderma*: Presence of internal organ involvement, Raynaud's phenomenon, abnormal nailfold capillaries and positive serology in the absence of skin sclerosis is termed as *SSc sine scleroderma*.
- *CREST*: *C*alcinosis, *R*aynaud's phenomenon, *E*sophageal dysmotility, *S*clerodactyly and *T*elangiectasias. This acronym is used sometimes for a subset of limited SSc patients with these specific features.

A dermatologist's role in early diagnosis of the disease is of significance because of the high morbidity as well as mortality.

8.2 Pathogenesis [1]

It is an interplay of three main factors as depicted in Fig. 8.1.

Role of B cells- Though systemic sclerosis is mediated mainly through inflammatory mediators secreted from the T cells, B cells also appear to affect the fibrosis in a number of ways. They seem to stimulate the fibroblasts through autoantibodies, by contact-dependent mechanism and through production of profibrotic cytokines.

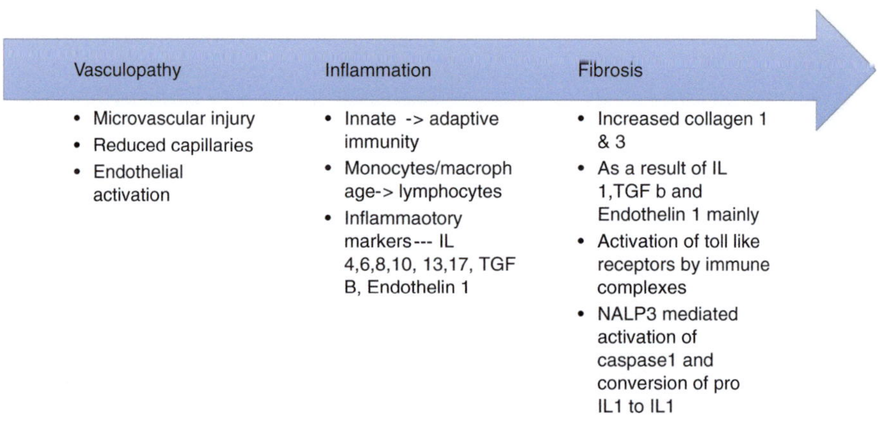

Fig. 8.1 Pathogenesis of systemic sclerosis

8.3 Cutaneous Features [2, 3]

There are three ill-defined phases of the disease (Fig. 8.2), and a patient usually presents in the indurated stage to a dermatologist.

8.3.1 Raynaud's Phenomenon

It is usually the earliest symptom to develop. Typical triphasic colour changes (Pallor–cyanosis–rubor) may not be appreciated in every case, and only biphasic changes may be noted. Initially it occurs only in winters, but slowly episodes may occur after even minute exposure to cold in summer season also as the disease progresses. Secondary changes like digital ulcerations, pitted scars and loss of pulp of digits develop over the years and are seen more commonly in limited SSc.

8.3.2 Face (Fig. 8.3)

- Loss of wrinkles and expressions due to tautness of skin giving rise to mask-like facies.
- Beaking/narrowing of nose.
- Mat-like telangiectasis over cheeks.
  - Common over cheeks, lips, palms.
  - Marker for vasculopathy.
  - Occult or potential development of PAH.

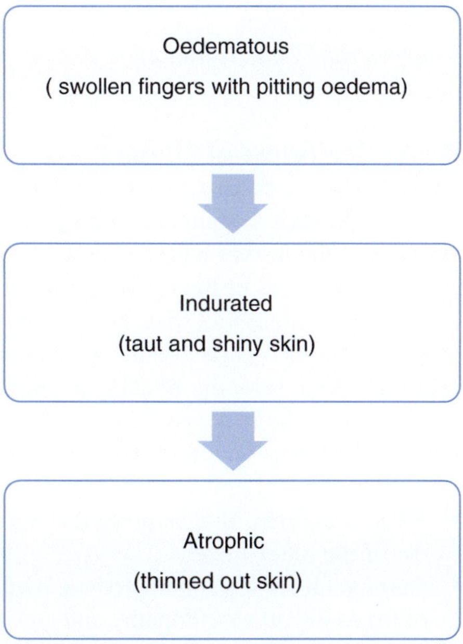

Fig. 8.2 Stages of systemic sclerosis

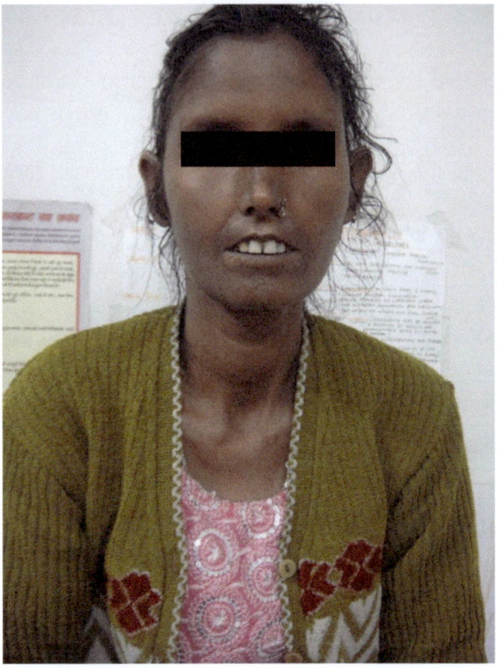

Fig. 8.3 Typical facial appearance in systemic sclerosis

- Inability to pull down the lower eyelid—*Ingram sign.*
- Perioral radial furrowing (purse string appearance) along with restricted mouth opening (microstomia).
- Loss of buccal pad of fat giving a narrowed appearance to face with prominent zygomatic bones.
- Dyschromic pigmentation over face.

8.3.3 Puffiness of Fingers

It is seen in early oedematous phase of the disease which may be associated with stiffness of the fingers with decreased functional ability (Fig. 8.4).

In initial stages of the disease, pulp of the fingers becomes swollen (*round pad sign/Mizutani sign*), but over the course, the pulp of fingers is lost, and the fingers taper to give the characteristic appearance of sclerodactyly. In late stages, due to sclerosis of the skin, the fingers become fixed in a semi-flexed position. Gangrene of digits may also be seen in many cases. There may be ulcers present over the digital tips which heal leaving behind pitted scars (Fig. 8.5).

- Pitted scars may also be present along the ulnar border of thumb and radial border of the index finger.
- Chronic ulcers with characteristic burning sensation may develop over the dorsa of limbs due to vasculopathy and add to morbidity of the patient.

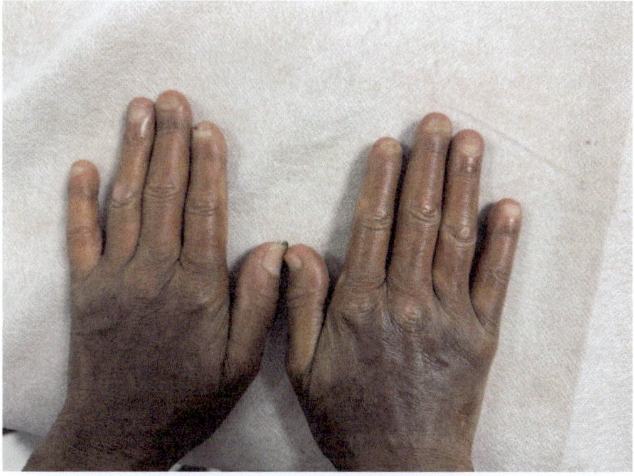

Fig. 8.4 Swollen fingers in initial stage of systemic sclerosis

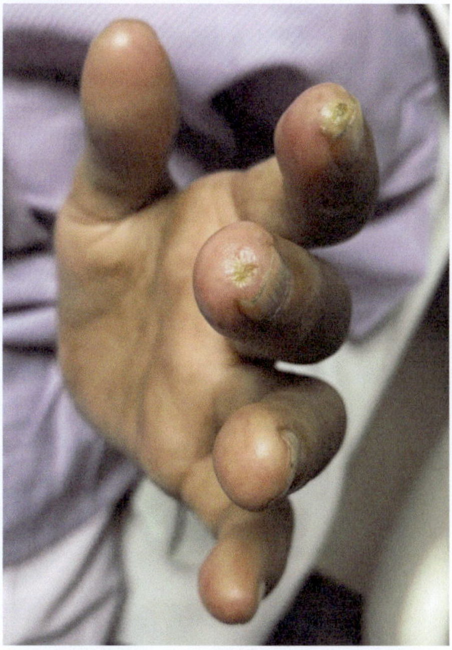

Fig. 8.5 Digital pitted scars

- *Pterygium inversum unguis* or *ventral pterygium*, the adherence of the distal portion of the nailbed to the ventral surface of the nail plate can be seen. It is commonly seen with systemic sclerosis and some time with systemic lupus erythematosus.

8.3.4 Skin Thickening

The characteristic skin thickening develops later and is often complained by the patient as a feeling of tightness, inability to pinch the skin over affected part and difficulty in opening the mouth. The extent of skin tightness is the deciding factor for the classification of the disease into its two subsets: limited and diffuse SSc. Involvement of the skin above the elbows/knees and trunk hails a poorer prognosis and is classified as diffuse SSc.

In diffuse SSc, bound-down skin along with pigmentary changes is seen over the trunk. There is tightening of the skin of the neck which becomes more evident on neck extension (*Barnett neck sign*). There may loss of sweating with diminished hair on the sclerotic skin.

Cobble stone appearance of hidebound skin may be seen due to lymphangiectasias.

8.3.5 Pigmentation of Skin

Various types of pigmentary changes which have been seen in SSc include:

- Diffuse generalized pigmentation (mimicking Addison's disease).
- Localized hyperpigmentation over areas of sclerosis.
- *Leucoderma of scleroderma* which is focal depigmentation with sparing of perifollicular pigmentation (salt and pepper sign). It favours the upper trunk, face and limbs (Fig. 8.6).
- Streaky pigmentation over blood vessels.
- Reticulate hyperpigmentation.
- Dense warty pigmentation in flexures (mimicking Acanthosis nigricans).
  - Proposed hypotheses for pigmentary changes include increased endothelin 1 mediated melanin synthesis, increased production of melanocyte growth factors by fibroblasts and a possible thermoregulatory mechanism.

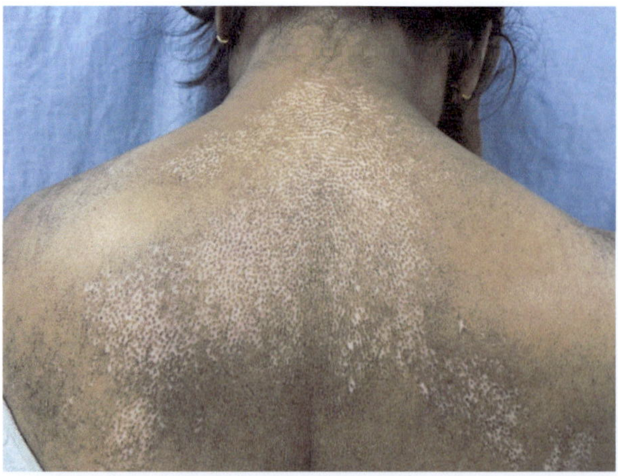

Fig. 8.6 Salt and pepper pigmentation over the trunk

8.3.6 Scalp

Diffuse thinning of hair may be seen.

8.3.7 Calcinosis

Calcinosis with painful hard nodules is seen over the fingers and joints, more commonly in limited SSc. Rarely, nodules can be seen over the face also (Fig. 8.7). They rupture to discharge chalky white material and leave atrophic scars.

8.3.8 Nails

Lustreless with ragged cuticles and increased curvature as a result of the loss of pulp can be seen. Nailfold capillaroscopy findings are described in a separate chapter.

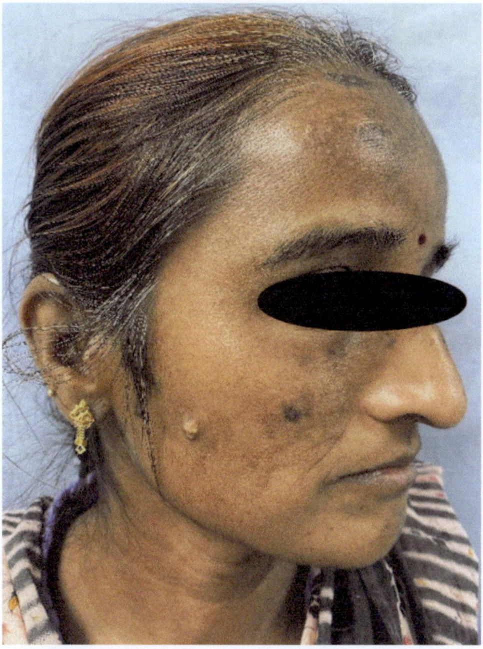

Fig. 8.7 Calcinosis cutis over face

8.4 Systemic Manifestations [4, 5]

8.4.1 Gastrointestinal Symptoms

They occur early and may be overlooked or treated by over-the-counter medicines by the patients themselves. Oesophageal involvement occurs in 90% cases and is more significant in limited SSc (Fig. 8.8).

- *Pseudo-obstruction* with colicky abdominal pain and volvulus may also occur. In rare cases, *pneumatosis cystoides intestinalis* may occur in the small intestine and presents with recurrent intestinal obstruction or pneumoperitoneum as a result of cyst rupture.
- *Telangiectasias*: They may occur in any part of the gastrointestinal tract leading to bleeding, most commonly in the stomach (gastric antral vascular ectasia/GAVE).

8.4.2 Pulmonary Involvement

Pulmonary involvement occurs in the form of interstitial lung disease (ILD), idiopathic pulmonary fibrosis and pulmonary artery hypertension (PAH).

- Currently the leading cause of mortality in SSc.
- Breathlessness is one of the early symptoms and may be accompanied by dry cough, palpitations and peripheral oedema.

8.4.3 Cardiac Involvement

Cardiac involvement is in the form of myositis and arrhythmias.

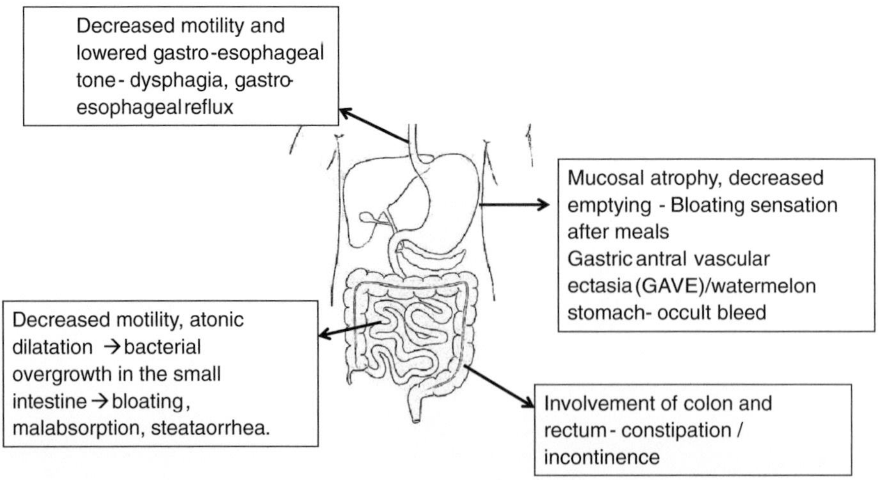

Fig. 8.8 Pictorial depiction of gastrointestinal involvement with common symptoms

8.4.4 Scleroderma Renal Crisis (SRC)

Scleroderma renal crisis (SRC) is the most serious complication of SSc. The incidence and mortality have declined recently due to early use of ACE inhibitors in the treatment. Risk factors for SRC are summarized in Table 8.1. A stable SSc patient who abruptly develops acute renal failure with or without accelerated hypertension and symptoms of headaches, visual disturbances and congestive heart failure should be considered as a medical emergency and managed judiciously.

8.4.5 Musculoskeletal Involvement

Low-grade myopathy with mild derangement of creatine kinase or mildly abnormal electromyogram may also occur. This is opposed to the inflammatory myositis which may be seen in cases with overlap where laboratory abnormalities are more pronounced. Radiological changes in the skeletal involvement include:

- Terminal resorption of digits.
- Calcinosis (differentiates from RP which may have terminal resorption in late cases).
- Erosive arthropathy giving pestle and mortar appearance.
- Increased intraosseous calcium deposition.
- Osteopoikilosis.
- Tendon friction rubs: Felt as coarse crepitus like sensation over the wrist/elbow/ankle/knee joints and are seen more commonly in diffuse SSc and herald a poorer prognosis.

8.4.6 Rarely Affected Systems

- Dental—Thickening and widening of periodontal membrane *(Stafne's sign).*
- Central nervous system—Neuropathy may occur in less than 10% cases.

Table 8.1 Risk factors for scleroderma renal crisis

Clinical	Male gender, early diffuse cutaneous SSc (< 4 years), rapid and extensive thickening of skin, tendon friction rubs, large joint contractures due to skin tightening, myopathy, cardiovascular pathology
Drugs	Prednisolone dose ≥ 15 mg/d/low dose for long duration, cyclosporine, tacrolimus
Autoantibodies	Anti-RNA polymerase III antibody

Table 8.2 Differentiation between limited and diffuse SSc

Features	Limited SSc (lSSc)	Diffuse SSc (dSSc)
Extent of skin involvement	Limited to distal extremities and sometimes face	Involvement of proximal extremities, trunk and face
Duration of Raynaud's phenomenon	Long	Short (<1 year)
Onset and progress of skin tightening	Slow	Rapid
Clinical features Calcinosis Telangiectasias Tendon friction rubs Musculoskeletal features Nailfold capillaroscopy	More common More common Less common Less common Capillary dilatation	Less common Less common More common More common Capillary dropouts
Internal organ involvement Oesophageal dysmotility Pulmonary Renal Cardiomyopathy	Late onset More common PAH > ILD Low risk of renal crises Less common	Early onset Less common ILD > PAH High risk of renal crises More common
Autoantibodies Anticentromere Antitopoisomerase (Scl-70) Anti-RNA polymerase III	+ in 40–50% + in 0–5% Usually negative	+ in 0–5% + in 0–20% + in 10%
Prognosis	More favourable	Less favourable

8.5 Limited Versus Diffuse Cutaneous Systemic Sclerosis [6, 7]

The two major subtypes, limited and diffuse cutaneous systemic sclerosis, can be differentiated further with the help of certain other features (Table 8.2).

8.6 Diagnostic Criteria [8]

The earliest criteria were suggested in 1980 by the American College of Rheumatology (ACR) and were developed after evaluating patients who had long-standing SSc. They are known as *Preliminary criteria for the classification of systemic sclerosis (scleroderma)* and have one major and three minor criteria.

Major
Proximal scleroderma.

Minor
1. Sclerodactyly.
2. Digital pitted scars or loss of substance from the finger pads.
3. Bibasilar pulmonary fibrosis.

Table 8.3 ACR/EULAR criteria for SSc

Feature	Subfeature	Score
Skin thickening of the fingers (extending proximal to the MCP joints)	*Sufficient criteria*	9
Skin thickening of the fingers	Puffy fingers Whole finger, distal to MCP	2 4
Fingertip lesions Telangiectasia Abnormal nailfold capillaries Raynaud's phenomenon Pulmonary artery hypertension and/or interstitial lung disease SSc-related autoantibodies (any of anticentromere/anti Scl-70/ anti-RNA polymerase III)	Digital tip ulcers Pitting scars	2 3 2 2 3 2 3
Add the maximum score in each category. Score 9 or more classifies the patient as SSc		

One major or two or more minor criteria are needed for the diagnosis of SSc.

But these criteria had low sensitivity especially in cases with limited SSc or shorter duration disease, often resulting in exclusion of around 20% patients with limited SSc from clinical studies.

In 2013, ACR and the European League Against Rheumatism (EULAR) established the latest criteria (ACR/EULAR criteria) which have the advantage of better sensitivity and specificity than all the previous criteria [3]. The three hallmarks of SSc, fibrosis of skin and/or internal organs, vasculopathy and SSc-specific autoantibodies, all are included in this. A point system is applied to the various manifestations and maximum score is calculated. Thickening of the skin of the fingers proximal to the metacarpophalangeal joints constitutes the single sufficient criteria to classify a patient as SSc. But if this is not fulfilled, then the maximum score is calculated by adding the highest points in each category, and patients with 9 or more points are classified as having SSc (Table 8.3).

However, it is stressed that they are mainly intended to include the patients in clinical trials by dermatologists/rheumatologists/researchers and not for diagnosis of SSc. The diagnosis of SSc still remains more of a clinical judgement as many features like dysphagia/calcinosis/tendon friction rubs which may suggest the diagnosis have not been included in the criteria. Moreover, they are inapplicable in patients who have a SSc-like disorder such as nephrogenic sclerosing fibrosis, graft versus host disease, generalized morphea, eosinophilic fasciitis, scleredema diabeticorum, scleromyxedema, etc. and in patients who have *skin thickening sparing the fingers*.

Prescleroderma and VEDOSS (Very Early Diagnosis of Systemic Sclerosis) Criteria for the Diagnosis [9]

A subset of disease is being identified which has Raynaud's phenomenon along with nailfold capillaroscopic changes and autoantibodies in absence of any evident skin thickening. It is thought to be a very early stage of systemic sclerosis 'prescleroderma', and further research is ongoing.

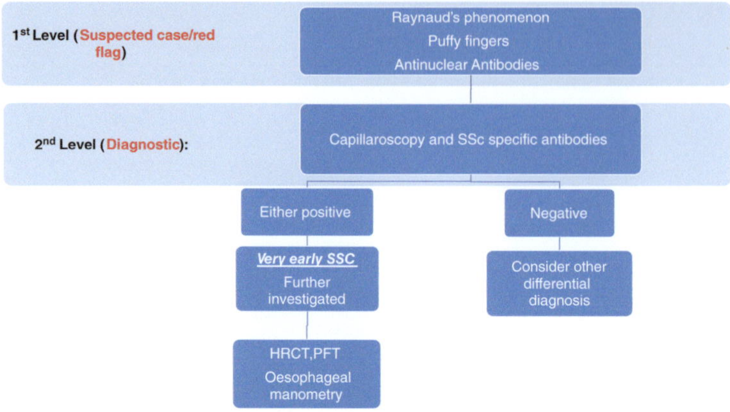

Fig. 8.9 Criteria for very early diagnosis of systemic sclerosis (VEDOSS)

These criteria help to identify very early scleroderma before the actual involvement of the skin (Fig. 8.9).

8.7 Severity Assessment [10, 11]

- Modified Rodnan Skin Scoring system (mRSS): It is the most commonly used method to assess the skin tightening as it can be done in a few minutes and is non-invasive. The degree of skin sclerosis is scored from 0 to 3 at 17 body sites, and a maximum score of 51 can be seen (Fig. 8.10). It has been established that mRSS correlates well with the disease process and may serve as a surrogate marker for the degree of internal organ involvement and disease outcome. Disadvantages include lack of objectivity, inter-observer variations and less sensitivity in early disease with small degrees of skin thickening.
- 20 mHz USG. When done with technically sound methods, high-frequency USG has an advantage of assessing the skin thickness properly as it is easily able to differentiate the layers of skin as epidermis, dermis and subcutaneous tissue. The skin thickness as well as dermal oedema can be studied, and the results have been seen to correlate with mRSS.
- Optical coherence tomography—it is a latest imaging technique and shows reduction in optical density of papillary dermis which histopathologically correlates with the dermal fibrosis.

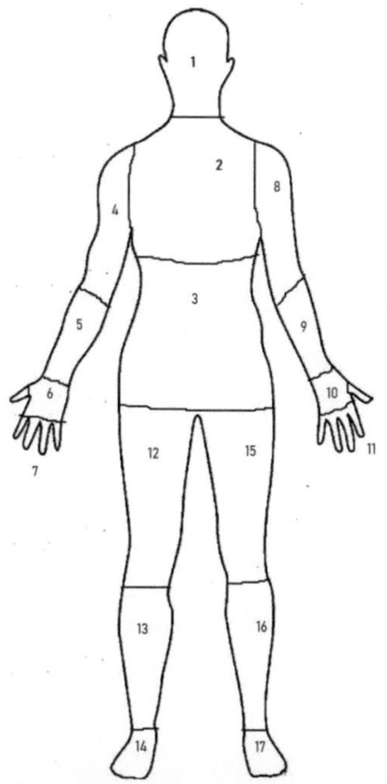

17 Sites

Face

Chest

Abdomen

Upper arm – right and left

Forearm – right and left

Hands– right and left

Fingers– right and left

Thighs– right and left

Legs– right and left

Foot – right and left

(The numbers given in the diagram are only for pictorial depiction and ease of calculation)

Scoring

0- Normal

1- Possible thickening

2- Unable to pinch the skin

3- Unable to move the skin(fixed to deeper tissues)

Fig. 8.10 Pictorial depiction of mRSS

8.8 Complications [12]

It goes without saying that AI-CTD should always be managed in conjunction with a rheumatologist. A dermatologist also should be aware of certain imminent conditions which should always be looked at the time of follow-up visits for timely referral to specialists.

- SRC is the most dreaded complication; hence regular monitoring of blood pressure is necessary along with periodic renal function tests. Any sign suggestive of progressive hypertension with decreased renal function warrants timely nephrologist opinion.
- Pulmonary manifestations may progress slowly, but history of progressive increase in cough, breathlessness and syncope needs expert pulmonologist opinion.

8.9 Prognosis [13–15]

Poor prognosis is seen in the following:

- Males.
- Extensive cutaneous involvement.
- Low systolic BP.
- Reduction of DLCO to <40%.
- Tendon friction rubs.
- High mean right atrial pressure.
- Reduced 6-minute walk distance (marker of cardiorespiratory severity).

8.10 Differential Diagnosis [16]

There are many diseases which mimic SSc and can be broadly classified as localized or systemic disorders which have tightness of the skin as one of the presenting features (Fig. 8.11). A physician should be aware of these conditions to overcome clinical over-diagnosis of SSc.

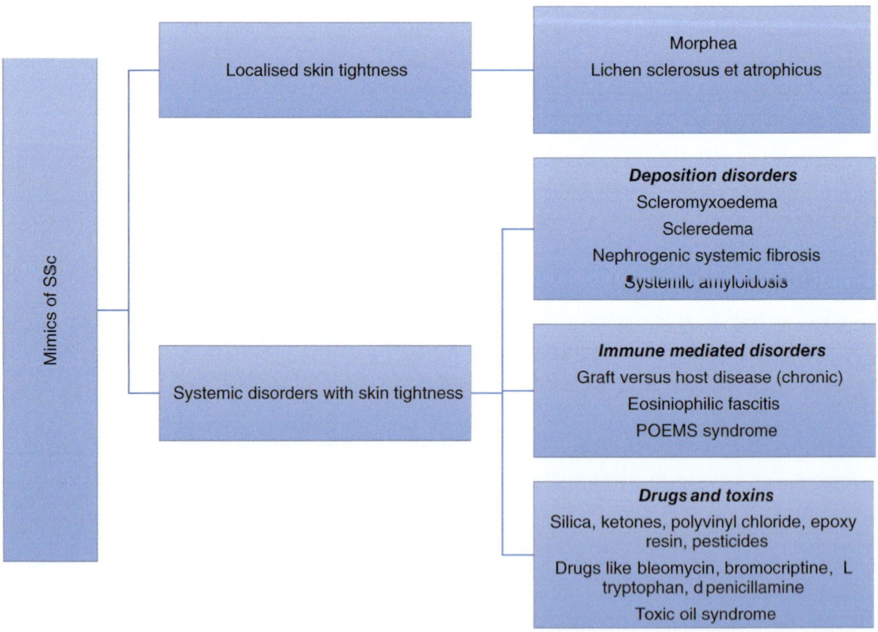

Fig. 8.11 Scleroderma mimics

8.11 Conclusion

Systemic sclerosis exemplifies the complex interplay between immune activation, vascular injury and progressive fibrosis, which ultimately results in a disease which has substantial clinical complexity and variability. Early identification of disease remains important to optimizing patient outcomes, as delays in diagnosis are associated with irreversible systemic involvement leading to increased mortality. A dermatologist's role is of paramount importance for the same. Diagnosis is usually clinical according to the latest EULAR criteria. Different autoantibodies are associated with the two different types of disease-limited and diffuse cutaneous systemic sclerosis, though some overlap may be there. Internal organ involvement in the form of cardiac and pulmonary systems is the most common cause of morbidity as well as mortality.

References

1. Rosendahl AH, Schönborn K, Krieg T. Pathophysiology of systemic sclerosis (scleroderma). Kaohsiung J Med Sci. 2022;38(3):187–95.
2. Lescoat A, Huang S, Carreira PE, et al. Cutaneous manifestations, clinical characteristics, and prognosis of patients with systemic sclerosis sine scleroderma: data from the international EUSTAR database. JAMA Dermatol. 2023;159(8):837–47. https://doi.org/10.1001/jamadermatol.2023.1729.
3. Chuamanochan M, Haws AL, Pattanaprichakul P. Reticulate hyperpigmentation in systemic sclerosis: a case report and review of the literature. J Med Case Rep. 2015;9:219.
4. Pearson DR, Werth VP, Pappas-Taffer L. Systemic sclerosis: current concepts of skin and systemic manifestations. Clin Dermatol. 2018;36(4):459–74. https://doi.org/10.1016/j.clindermatol.2018.04.004.
5. Foocharoen C, Tonsawan P, Pongkulkiat P, Anutrakulchai S, Mahakkanukrauh A, Suwannaroj S. Management review of scleroderma renal crisis: an update with practical pointers. Mod Rheumatol. 2023;33(1):12–20.
6. Ostojić P, Damjanov N. Different clinical features in patients with limited and diffuse cutaneous systemic sclerosis. Clin Rheumatol. 2006;25:453–7. https://doi.org/10.1007/s10067-005-0041-0.
7. Van Den Hoogen F, Khanna D, Fransen J, Johnson SR, Baron M, Tyndall A, Matucci-Cerinic M, Naden RP, Medsger TA Jr, Carreira PE, Riemekasten G. 2013 classification criteria for systemic sclerosis: an American College of Rheumatology/European league against rheumatism collaborative initiative. Arthritis Rheum. 2013;65(11):2737–47.
8. Volkmann ER, Andréasson K, Smith V. Systemic sclerosis. Lancet. 2023;401(10373):304–18.
9. Avouac J, Fransen J, Walker UA, et al. Preliminary criteria for the very early diagnosis of systemic sclerosis: results of a Delphi consensus study from EULAR scleroderma trials and research group. Ann Rheum Dis. 2011;70(3):476–81.
10. Kumánovics G, Péntek M, Bae S, Opris D, Khanna D, Furst DE, Czirják L. Assessment of skin involvement in systemic sclerosis. Rheumatology. 2017;56(suppl_5):v53–66. https://doi.org/10.1093/rheumatology/kex202.
11. Matsuda KM, Yoshizaki A, Kuzumi A, Fukasawa T, Ebata S, Miura S, Toyama T, Yoshizaki A, Sumida H, Asano Y, Oba K. Skin thickness score as a surrogate marker of organ involvements in systemic sclerosis: a retrospective observational study. Arthritis Res Ther. 2019;21:10.
12. Allanore Y, Simms R, Distler O, Trojanowska M, Pope J, Denton CP, Varga J. Systemic sclerosis. Nat Rev Dis Primers. 2015;1(1):1–21.

13. Pokeerbux MR, Giovannelli J, Dauchet L, et al. Survival and prognosis factors in systemic sclerosis: data of a French multicenter cohort, systematic review, and meta-analysis of the literature. Arthritis Res Ther. 2019;21:86. https://doi.org/10.1186/s13075-019-1867-1.
14. Doré A, Lucas M, Ivanco D, Medsger TA Jr, Domsic RT. Significance of palpable tendon friction rubs in early diffuse cutaneous systemic sclerosis. Arthritis Care Res (Hoboken). 2013;65(8):1385–9. https://doi.org/10.1002/acr.21964.
15. Sanges S, Giovannelli J, Sobanski V, Morell-Dubois S, Maillard H, Lambert M, Podevin C, Lamblin N, De Groote P, Bervar JF, Perez T, Matran R, Rémy-Jardin M, Hatron PY, Hachulla É, Launay D. Factors associated with the 6-minute walk distance in patients with systemic sclerosis. Arthritis Res Ther. 2017;19(1):279. https://doi.org/10.1186/s13075-017-1489-4.
16. Ferreli C, Gasparini G, Parodi A, Cozzani E, Rongioletti F, Atzori L. Cutaneous manifestations of scleroderma and scleroderma-like disorders: a comprehensive review. Clin Rev Allergy Immunol. 2017;53(3):306–36.

Morphea

9

Sudip Ghosh, Sharmistha Panja, and Partha Mukherjee

Abstract

Morphea is a chronic inflammatory disorder characterized by localized skin and subcutaneous sclerosis, with potential extracutaneous involvement in up to 25% of cases. The disease exhibits a broad clinical spectrum, from isolated plaques to severe, generalized forms leading to disfigurement and functional impairment. Clinically, morphea presents with progressive skin thickening, pigmentary changes, and, in some cases, musculoskeletal, neurological, ocular, and oral complications. The German classification system categorizes it into various subtypes, including circumscribed, generalized, and linear morphea. Differential diagnoses depend on disease stage, with systemic sclerosis being a key exclusion.

Keywords

Skin thickening · Plaques · Atrophy · Morphea

9.1 Introduction

Morphea is a chronic, idiopathic inflammatory disorder characterized by skin sclerosis. It is usually confined to skin and subcutaneous tissue, but extracutaneous manifestations are seen in up to 25% of patients approximately. The disease has a heterogeneous spectrum of presentations ranging from localized solitary plaques to

S. Ghosh (✉) · S. Panja
Department of Dermatology, Venereology, & Leprosy, R.G. Kar Medical College, Kolkata, West Bengal, India

P. Mukherjee
Department of Dermatology, Venereology, & Leprosy, College of Medicine & JNM Hospital, Kalyani, West Bengal, India

P. Agarwal et al. (eds.), *Dermatologist's Handbook of Autoimmune Connective Tissue Diseases*, https://doi.org/10.1007/978-981-95-0524-1_9

generalized involvement with associated severe disfigurement and compromised quality of life.

9.2 Pathogenesis

It is not clearly understood. Autoimmunity, genetics, and vascular dysfunction possibly play an important role in the pathogenesis with trauma, radiation, and medications acting as predisposing factors (Fig. 9.1). Morphea uniformly involves tissue derived from mesoderm [1]. The involvement of different alleles on MHC

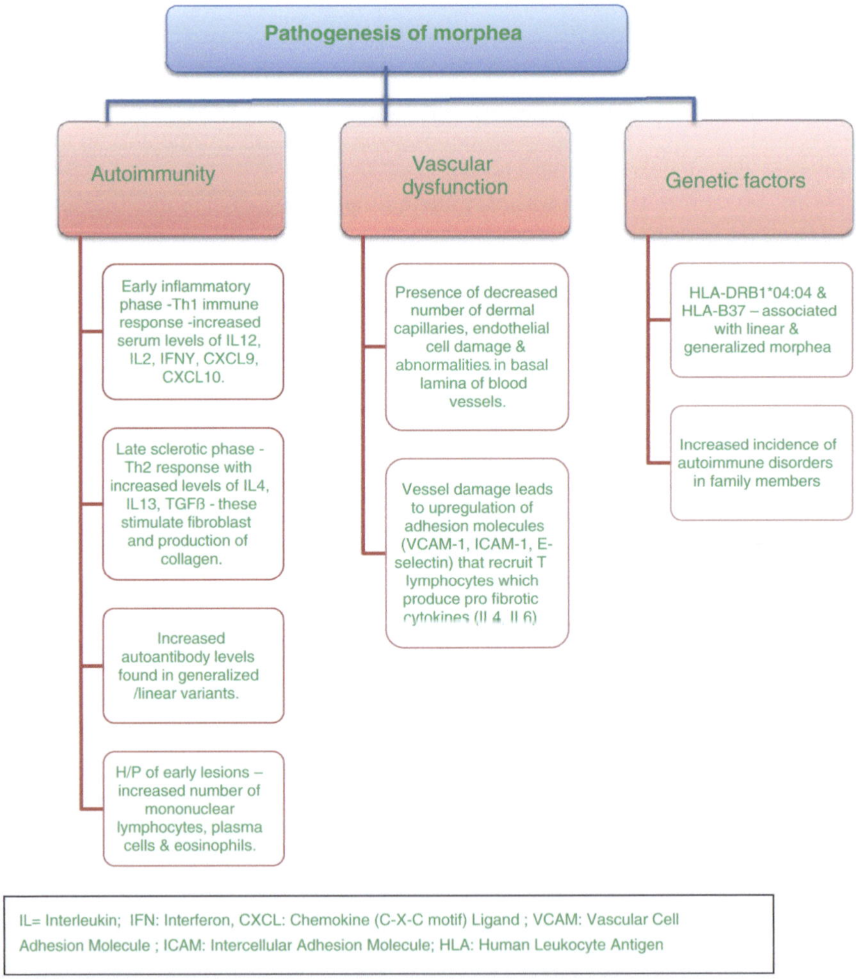

Fig. 9.1 Pathogenesis of morphea

(DRB1*04:04 and HLA-B*37) and cytokine profile (levels of IL-2 and IL-6 are raised more in morphea) has helped in understanding the difference between pathogenesis of morphea and systemic sclerosis [2].

9.3 Classifications

No universal classification exists. A simplified classification based on clinical phenotypes is given in Fig. 9.2 [3].

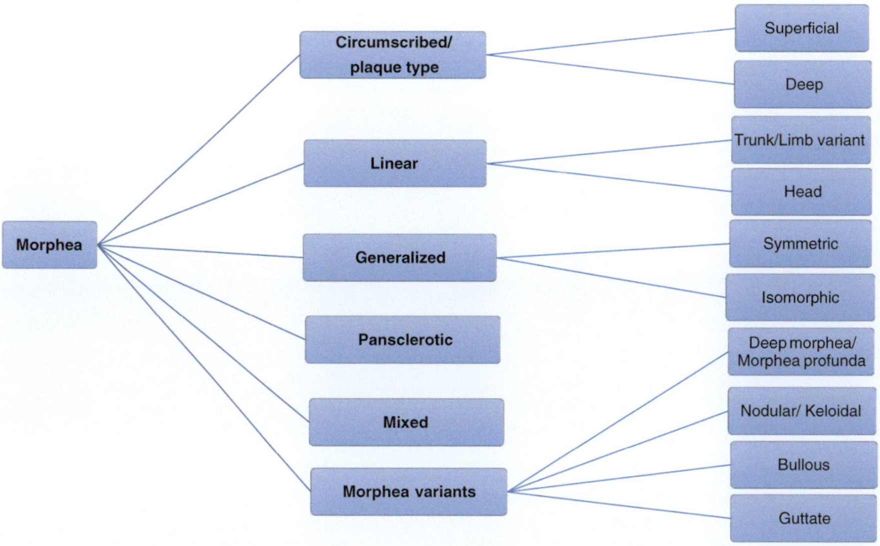

Fig. 9.2 Types of morphea

9.4 Clinical Features

Cutaneous

- It is usually asymptomatic.
- Changes in skin color and texture are usually the commonest presenting complaints.
  - Itching, pain, or numbness may rarely be present in actively inflamed areas.
- In the early stages, the lesions are better felt, hence need to be palpated to observe the thickening of skin than only inspection of lesion.
- One or more circumscribed patches of the skin with sclerotic changes in one anatomic site confined to the superficial panniculus (subcutaneous tissue) are termed as circumscribed type of morphea (Fig. 9.3), while four or more plaques that affect at least two anatomic sites are termed as generalized type [4].
- The presentation depends on the stage of development of the lesions (Fig. 9.4).

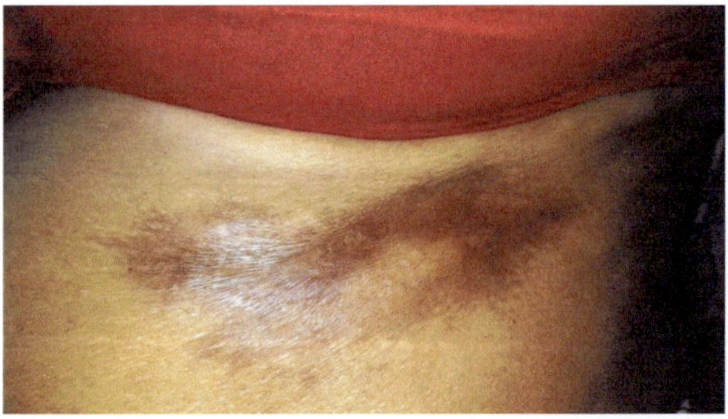

Fig. 9.3 Circumscribed morphea over the abdomen

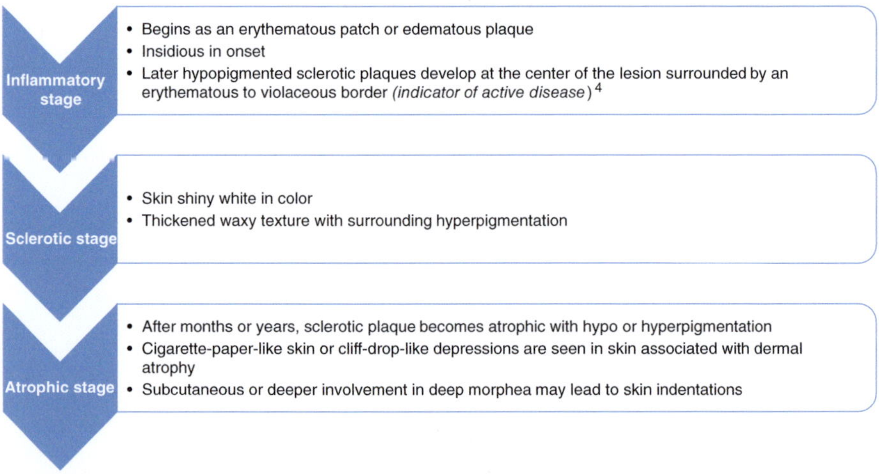

Fig. 9.4 Evolution of cutaneous lesions of morphea

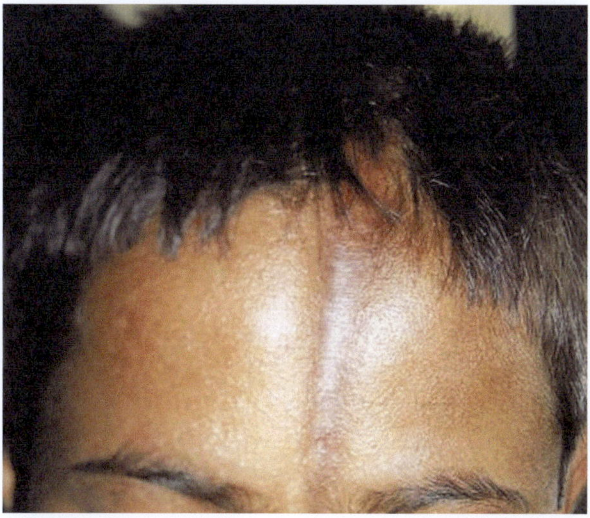

Fig. 9.5 En coup de sabre

- *Musculoskeletal*: Most common extracutaneous manifestation.
  - Arthralgia, joint swelling, myalgia, limb contracture, and limited range of motion.
  - Seen more in adults with generalized or deep morphea.
  - Disabling pansclerotic morphea is more commonly seen in children and causes lifelong disability due to involvement of underlying muscles and joint contractures [5].
- *Neurological*: It is mainly seen in children with linear morphea on the forehead (en coup de sabre) (Fig. 9.5).
  - Seizures (complex partial), headache, peripheral neuropathy, rarely cerebral vasculitis.
- *Ocular*: Eyes are rarely involved.
  - May have associated episcleritis, anterior uveitis, papilledema, glaucoma, refractory errors, eyelid, eyelash, and lacrimal gland abnormalities.
- *Oral and dental*: Involvement is seen only in cases with lesions over the face.
  - Malocclusion, overgrowth of the anterior lower third of the face, altered dentition, atrophy of salivary glands and tongue, and uvular deviation.

9.5 Differential Diagnosis

The differential diagnoses of morphea with respect to various clinical stages of involvement are enumerated in Table 9.1 [1]. Systemic sclerosis needs to be differentiated from generalized morphea, and the features are mentioned in Table 9.2.

Table 9.1 Differential diagnosis of morphea

Morphea subtypes	Differential diagnosis
Initial inflammatory phase	Lichen sclerosus (early lesions) Erythema chronicum migrans Cutaneous mastocytosis Granuloma annulare Mycosis fungoides (early lesions) Panniculitis Lupus profundus
Well-developed plaque form	Inflammatory vitiligo Morpheaform BCC
Late stage with post inflammatory hyperpigmentation	Post-inflammatory hyperpigmentation Actinic lichen planus Café au lait macules Erythema dyschromicum perstans
Late atrophic stage	Acrodermatitis chronica atrophicans Morpheaform sarcoidosis Lipodystrophy Lichen sclerosus (advanced lesions) Scarring
Late sclerotic stage	Necrobiosis lipoidica Pretibial myxedema Cutaneous metastasis
Generalized morphea	Systemic sclerosis Chronic graft versus host disease Nephrogenic systemic fibrosis Scleredema Scleromyxedema Porphyria cutanea tarda
Linear morphea (Fig. 9.6)	Localized lipodystrophy Focal dermal dysplasia Eosinophilic cellulitis Steroid-induced atrophy

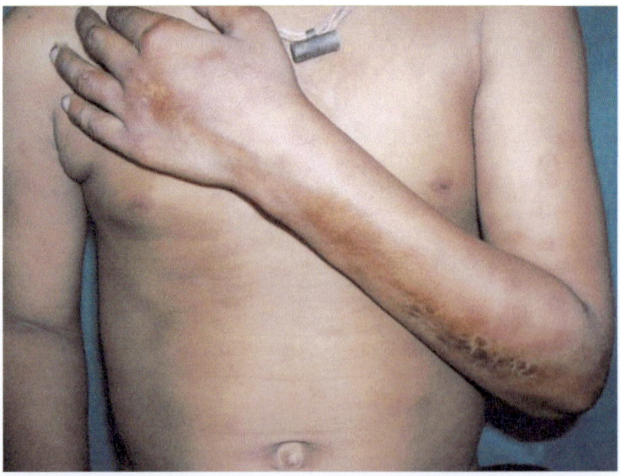

Fig. 9.6 Linear morphea on hand

Table 9.2 Differentiating features between generalized morphea and systemic sclerosis

Clinical and laboratory criteria	Systemic sclerosis	Morphea
Acral sclerosis/sclerodactyly	Present	Absent
Nailfold capillary changes	Present	Absent
Raynaud's phenomenon	Common	Extremely rare
Internal organ involvement (pulmonary, renal, GI)	Common	Very rare
Autoantibodies ANA	Present in >95%	Present in about 18–68%
Spontaneous remission	Does not occur	Can occur

9.6 Complications

- *Cutaneous*—facial atrophy, cicatricial alopecia (in en coup de sabre), facial deformity, bullae, ulcers following circumferential sclerosis of extremities.
- *Musculoskeletal*—limited motion range, limb-length discrepancy, joint deformity, joint contractures.
- *Malignancy*: Squamous cell carcinoma can develop in long-standing cases of pansclerotic morphea after 10–20 years.
- *Psychological*—negative effect on the quality of life.

9.7 Prognosis

- Rarely life-threatening.
- May be self-limited, but frequently remitting and relapsing course over several years.
- Recurrence occurs in 25% of patients. It is more common in linear limb variant of morphea (31%).

9.8 Conclusion

Morphea is a chronic inflammatory condition with a variable clinical spectrum ranging from isolated skin plaques to deep, disabling forms with extracutaneous involvement. Its pathogenesis is multifaceted. Early diagnosis based on clinical features and appropriate differentiation from mimickers like systemic sclerosis is essential for effective management. It may be self-limited, but frequently follows a remitting and relapsing course over several years, emphasizing the need for vigilant long-term care and tailored therapeutic strategies.

References

1. Papara C, De Luca DA, Bieber K, Vorobyev A, Ludwig RJ. Morphea: the 2023update. Front Med. 2023;10:1108623. https://doi.org/10.3389/fmed.2023.1108623.
2. Fett N. Scleroderma: nomenclature, etiology, pathogenesis, prognosis, and treatments: facts and controversies. Clin Dermatol. 2013;31(4):432–7.
3. Kreuter A, Krieg T, Worm M, Wenzel J, Gambichler T, Kuhn A, et al. Diagnosis and therapy of localized scleroderma. J Dtsch Dermatol Ges. 2009;7:S1–S12.
4. Careta MF, Romiti R. Localized scleroderma: clinical spectrum and therapeutic update. An Bras Dermatol. 2015;90:62–73.
5. Kim A, Marinkovich N, Vasquez R, Jacobe HT. Clinical features of patients with Morphea and the Pansclerotic subtype: a cross-sectional study from the Morphea in adults and children cohort. J Rheumatol. 2014;41:106–12.

Dermatomyositis

10

Bela Shah

Abstract

Dermatomyositis (DM) is an idiopathic chronic, inflammatory myopathy with characteristic cutaneous manifestations in addition to symmetrical proximal muscle weakness and systemic involvement. In addition to the classic presentation, variants such as amyopathic and hypomyopathic DM are also recognized. The pathogenesis is believed to be multifactorial with immune-mediated vasculopathy, genetic predisposition, and environmental triggers playing a crucial part. Cutaneous signs include heliotrope rash and Gottron's papules, confluent macular violaceous erythema, and rare findings such as mechanic's hands, ulcerations, and poikiloderma. Systemic involvement includes respiratory, cardiac, gastrointestinal, and musculoskeletal systems. Juvenile DM shows distinct clinical features including a higher incidence of calcinosis and lower malignancy risk. Diagnosis relies heavily on clinical acumen, and early recognition and intervention are essential to reduce morbidity and improve outcomes.

Keywords

Muscle weakness · Heliotrope rash · Confluent macular violaceous erythema · Calcinosis cutis

10.1 Introduction

Dermatomyositis (DM) is an autoimmune connective tissue disorder which predominantly affects the skin and skeletal muscles. Internal organs such as the lungs, heart, joints, and pharynx may also be involved by the autoimmune process. It is

B. Shah (✉)
Department of Skin & VD, GCS Medical College, Hospital and Research Centre, Ahmedabad, Gujarat, India

P. Agarwal et al. (eds.), *Dermatologist's Handbook of Autoimmune Connective Tissue Diseases*, https://doi.org/10.1007/978-981-95-0524-1_10

Table 10.1 Diagnostic criteria for polymyositis and dermatomyositis

Features	Polymyositis	Dermatomyositis
1. Symmetrical proximal muscle weakness 2. Muscle biopsy evidence of myositis 3. Elevation in serum skeletal muscle enzymes 4. Characteristic EMG pattern of myositis 5. Typical rash of dermatomyositis	Definitive: All of 1–4 Probable: Any 3 of 1–4 Possible: Any 2 of 1–4	Definitive: 5 plus any 3 of 1–4 Probable: 5 plus any 2 of 1–4 Possible: 5 plus any 1 of 1–4

classified with polymyositis and inclusion body myositis under the title of idiopathic inflammatory myopathies (IIMs) (Box 10.1).

Box 10.1: Classification of Idiopathic Inflammatory Myopathies
- Dermatomyositis
- Overlap myositis
- Immune mediated necrotising myopathy
- Sporadic inclusion body myositis
- Polymyositis

The differentiating features between polymyositis and dermatomyositis as suggested by Bohan and Peter are summarized in Table 10.1 [1].

Other than classic presentation with both muscular and cutaneous features, there can be two other presentations:

Amyopathic DM [2] (dermatomyositis sine myositis): The cutaneous manifestations have confirmed features suggestive of classic DM, but there is no proximal muscle weakness or raised muscle enzymes for 6 months or longer duration.

Hypomyopathic DM [2]. The condition shows signs of muscle inflammation in the absence of clinical muscle weakness, characterized by specific cutaneous findings, non-erosive bilateral polyarthritis, and subclinical elevations of muscle enzymes.

10.2 Pathogenesis [3]

It is believed to be a humorally mediated vasculopathic disease with an immune-mediated process triggered by external agents in genetically predisposed individuals (Table 10.2).

Table 10.2 Various causative factors associated with dermatomyositis

Genetics	HLA-DR3 and -B8 (juvenile DM) HLA-DR7 and -DRw53 (anti-Mi-2 antibodies) HLA-DR52 (anti-Jo-1 antibodies) HLA-B14 and -B40 (adults with dermatomyositis overlap)
Infectious agents	Picorna virus (substrate for aminoacyl-tRNA synthetases) *E. coli* Coxsackie virus Echovirus (in patients with hypogammaglobulinemia)
Drugs and vaccines	Hydroxyurea TNF-α inhibitors Lipid-lowering drugs (statins > gemfibrozil) NSAIDS (nonsteroidal anti-inflammatory drugs) Cyclophosphamide Checkpoint inhibitors (e.g. ipilimumab) D-penicillamine BCG vaccine

10.3 Clinical Features

10.3.1 Cutaneous Manifestations [4, 5]

Classic DM (CDM) presents with pathognomonic cutaneous findings and progressive, symmetric proximal muscle weakness. Cutaneous disease precedes the appearance of myositis by 3–6 months in 30–50% of patients, while 10% of patients present with muscle symptoms prior to the development of skin findings. The myriad dermatological manifestations are summarized in Table 10.3.

Table 10.3 Cutaneous manifestations of dermatomyositis

Pathognomonic cutaneous manifestations	
Heliotrope sign	Confluent pink-violaceous erythema involving the upper eyelids, at times accompanied with edema (Fig. 10.1)
Gottron's papules	Pink-violaceous papules on the dorsal hands, with a predilection for the skin overlying the metacarpophalangeal and interphalangeal joints (Fig. 10.2)
Characteristic cutaneous manifestations	
Confluent macular violaceous erythema (CMVE)	Lilac to violaceous colored rash. The color is due to displacement of dermal vasculature by the dermal edema. Based on the locations, it has been named as various signs
(a) V sign	CMVE over V area of neck or upper chest (Fig. 10.3)
(b) Shawl sign	CMVE over upper back (Fig. 10.4)
(c) Sleeve sign	CMVE over upper outer arms (Fig. 10.5)
(d) Holster sign	CMVE over of lateral thighs (Fig. 10.6)
Gottron sign	Erythematous to violaceous papules over elbows and/or knees
Poikiloderma	Telangiectatic erythema, epidermal atrophy, and dyspigmentation mainly in a photo-distributed pattern
Calcinosis cutis	Hard, irregular papules or nodules favoring sites of trauma (elbows/knees) with or without pain and limitation of function (Fig. 10.7) Indicator of delay in diagnosis or prolong duration, ongoing inflammation, delay in the institution of immunosuppression specially in juvenile dermatomyositis, ischemia, fingertip ulceration, and associated with antibodies against melanoma differentiation associated gene-5 (MDA-5) and nuclear matrix protein-2, antiPM/Scl antibodies [5]

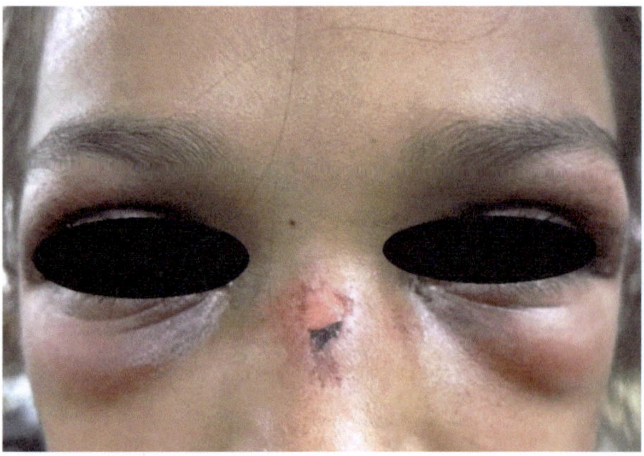

Fig. 10.1 Heliotrope rash—confluent pink-violaceous erythema and edema involving the eyelids

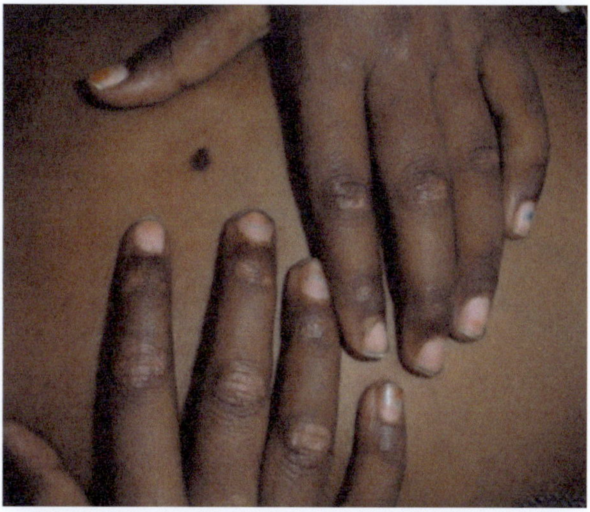

Fig. 10.2 Gottron papules—pink-violaceous papules on the skin overlying the metacarpophalangeal and interphalangeal joints

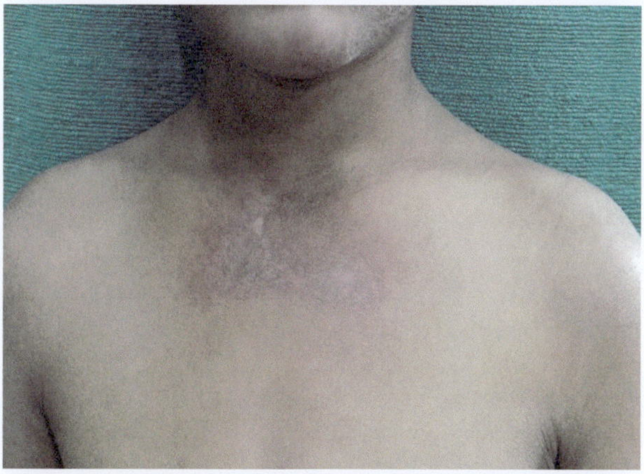

Fig. 10.3 V sign—confluent macular violaceous erythema over V area of the neck or upper chest

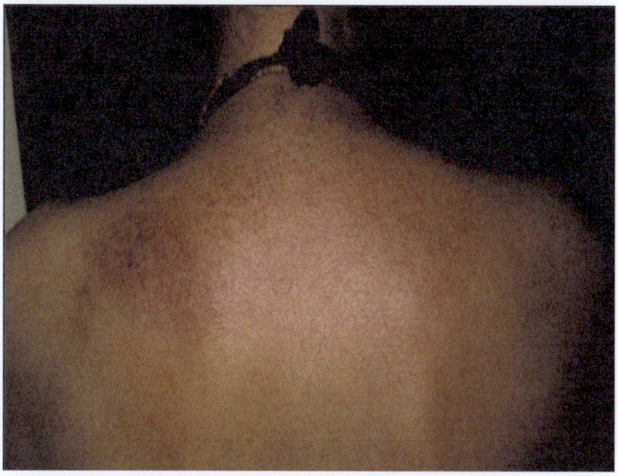

Fig. 10.4 Shawl sign—confluent macular violaceous erythema of the upper back

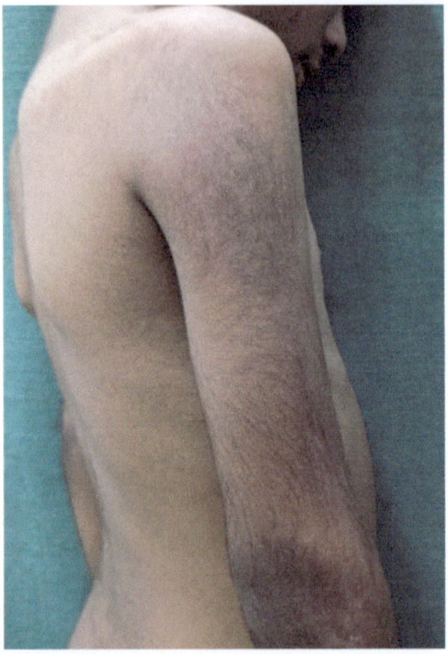

Fig. 10.5 Sleeve sign—confluent macular violaceous erythema over upper outer arms

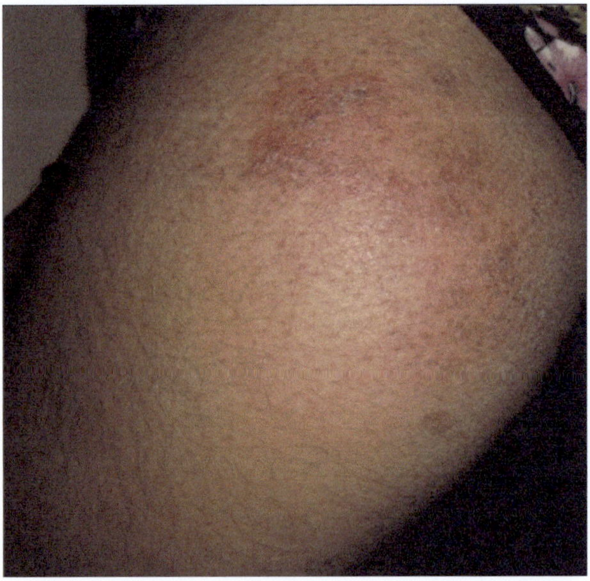

Fig. 10.6 Holster sign—confluent macular violaceous erythema CMVE over lateral thighs

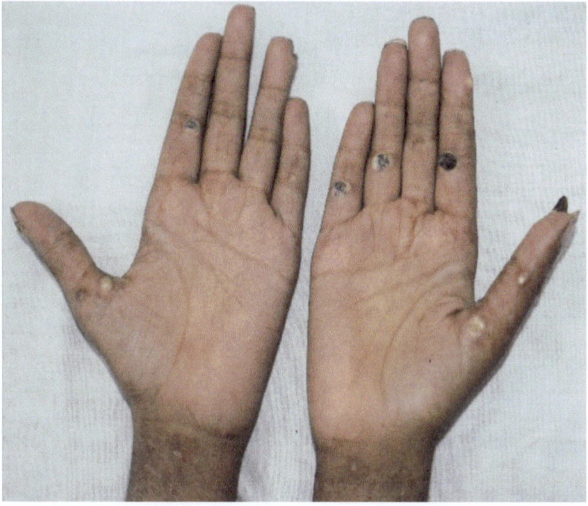

Fig. 10.7 Calcinosis cutis: hard, irregular papules, nodules over palm few having scab

10.3.2 Uncommon Presentations of Cutaneous Dermatomyositis [6, 7]

Besides the abovementioned hallmark cutaneous features, there are many clinical lesions which may be seen in DM:

- Cutaneous ulcerations or erosions. They can be a result of:
  - Vasculopathy.
  - Panniculitis.
  - Breakdown of poikilodermatous area.
  - Pressure from calcinosis.
- Mechanic's hands (antisynthetase syndrome): Thickening and roughness of the skin over the radial borders of fingers on palmar aspect. It is bilaterally symmetrical. Similar lesions may be seen on outer borders and planter aspect of feet **(Hiker's feet)** (Fig. 10.8).
- Tender palmar papules **(inverse Gottron's papules)**.
- Erythroderma.
- Cutaneous lesions that mimic pityriasis rubra pilaris **(Wong variant)**.
- Pustular eruption of the elbows and knees.
- Vesiculobullous lesions.
- Ovoid palatal patch (Fig. 10.9).
- Gingival telangiectasias.
- Flagellate erythema.
- Lipoatrophy (especially in juvenile DM).
- Small vessel vasculitis (especially in juvenile DM).
- **Samitz sign:** The sign refers to thickening, roughness, hyperkeratosis, and irregularity of the cuticle with minimum or no redness or inflammation.

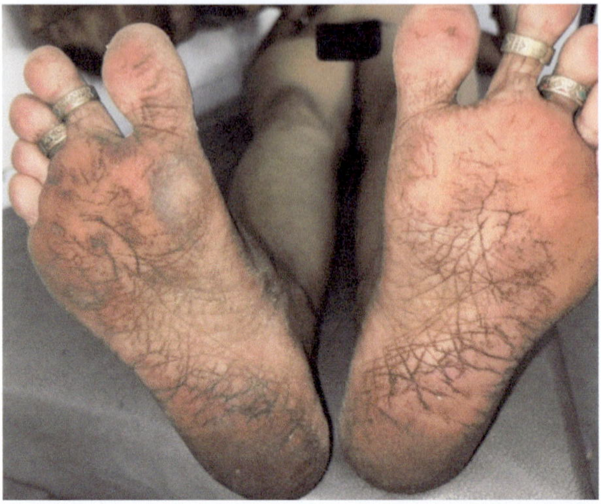

Fig. 10.8 Thickened skin over feet **(hiker's feet)**

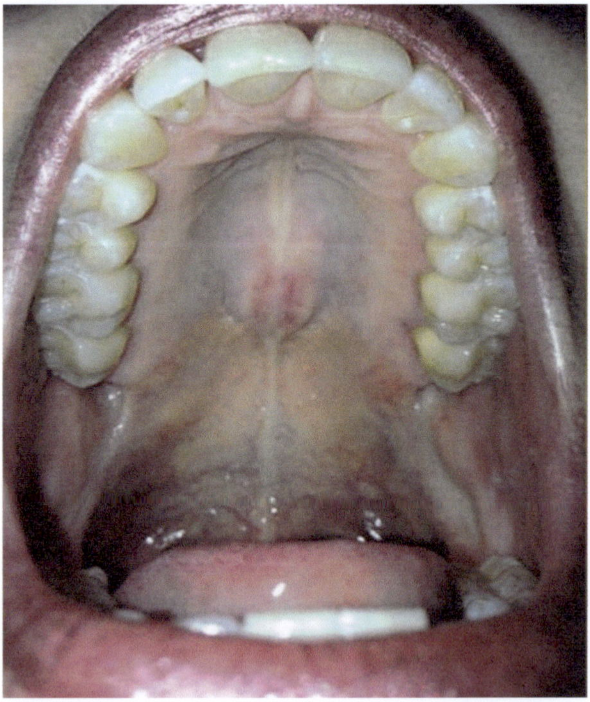

Fig. 10.9 Ovoid palatal patch

There is well-known association between malignancy and adult DM. The risk of association with malignancy increases with age, severe dermatological involvement with necrosis, diaphragmatic weakness, dysphagia, lack of interstitial lung disease, and presence of antibodies to anti-TIF1ɣ or NXP-2 (TIF, transcription intermediary factor; NXP, nuclear matrix protein). Most common cancers associated with DM are ovarian, colon, lung, breast, gastric, pancreatic, and lymphomas. A total of 80% of associated malignancies are adenocarcinomas.

10.3.3 Anti-synthetase Syndrome [8]

It is characterized by myositis, arthritis, fever, Raynaud's phenomenon, interstitial lung disease, and thickened skin over hands and feet (Fig. 10.8). The characteristic appearance of keratotic papules over borders of fingers gives the nomenclature **mechanic's hands**. It is associated with Anti Jo-1, Anti PL-7, Anti PL-12, IJ, and EJ autoantibodies.

10.4 Systemic Manifestations [9]

The Various Systemic Findings Seen in Dermatomyositis Are Summarized in Table 10.4.

Table 10.4 Systemic findings in DM

System affected	Clinical presentation	Secondary to
Musculoskeletal	Malaise Difficulty in combing hair or getting up from sitting position Difficulty in initiating swallowing Gastroesophageal reflux	Symmetric proximal muscle involvement, especially of the extensor groups (triceps and quadriceps Due to cricopharyngeal muscle dysfunction or possible overlap with systemic sclerosis Due to distal esophageal muscle involvement
Respiratory	Dry cough and progressive breathlessness	Diffuse interstitial fibrosis Acute respiratory distress syndrome
Cardiac	Chest pain, palpitations	Arrhythmias and conduction abnormalities
Joint	Multiple joint pain and swelling	Non-erosive inflammatory polyarthritis

10.5 Juvenile DM and Adult DM

Differences Between Juvenile Dermatomysitis and Adult Dermatomyositis Are Highlighted in Table 10.5.

Table 10.5 Differences between juvenile dermatomysitis and adult dermatomyositis

Juvenile dermatomyositis	Adult dermatomyositis
Most common idiopathic inflammatory myopathy	Polymyositis is more common than DM
Rash: Atypical, can occur anywhere in the body Ulcerative changes frequently seen	*Rash*: Typical of DM Ulcerative changes seen less frequently
Pulmonary involvement: Less common	*Pulmonary involvement*: More common
Malignancy risk: Low	*Malignancy risk*: High
Calcinosis: More common	*Calcinosis*: Less common
Anti-p155/140: Most common antibody	Anti Mi2: Most common antibody

10.6 Diagnosis

Given DM's protean manifestations, a detailed physical exam is at the cornerstone of making the correct diagnosis. Expert clinicians can usually arrive at a correct diagnosis of DM with a physical exam alone. When evaluating muscle disease, a detailed history with pointed questions (difficulty combing hair, getting out of a seated position, difficulty swallowing, change in voice) and strength testing of muscle groups should be performed at each clinic visit.

Sontheimer proposed the following diagnostic criteria for cutaneous dermatomyositis (Table 10.6).

The latest EULAR criteria for classification of inflammatory myopathies are given in Table 10.7.

Table 10.6 Criteria for diagnosis of DM

Major criteria
Heliotrope sign
Gottron's papules
Gottron sign
Minor criteria
Macular violaceous erythema involving (each area counts as a minor criterion) Scalp/anterior hairline Malar eminences of face, forehead, or chin V area of neck or upper chest (V sign) Posterior neck or posterior shoulders (shawl sign) Extensor surfaces of arms or forearms Linear streaking overlying extensor tendons of dorsal hands Periungual skin Lateral thighs or hips (holster sign) Medial malleoli
Nailfold capillary telangiectasia, hemorrhage-infarct
Poikiloderma
Mechanic's hands
Calcinosis cutis
Cutaneous ulcers
Pruritus
Dermatomyositis is diagnosed in presence of *Presence of* *Two major criteria or* *One major and two minor criteria* ***and*** *Skin biopsy changes consistent with cutaneous dermatomyositis*

Table 10.7 EULAR/ACR classification criteria for inflammatory myopathies

When no better explanation for the symptoms and signs exists, these classification criteria can be used			
Variable	Score points		
	Without muscle biopsy	With muscle biopsy	Definition
Age of onset			
Age of onset of first symptom assumed to be related to the disease ≥18 years and < 40 years	1.3	1.5	18 ≤ age (years) at onset of first symptom assumed to be related to the disease <40
Age of onset of first symptom assumed to be related to the disease ≥40 years	2.1	2.2	Age (years) at onset of first symptom assumed to be related to the disease ≥40
Muscle weakness			
Objective symmetric weakness, usually progressive, of the proximal upper extremities	0.7	0.7	Weakness of proximal upper extremities as defined by manual muscle testing or other objective strength testing, which is present on both sides and is usually progressive over time
Objective symmetric weakness, usually progressive, of the proximal lower extremities	0.8	0.5	Weakness of proximal lower extremities as defined by manual muscle testing or other objective strength testing, which is present on both sides and is usually progressive over time
Neck flexors are relatively weaker than neck extensors	1.9	1.6	Muscle grades for neck flexors are relatively lower than neck extensors as defined by manual muscle testing or other objective strength testing
In the legs proximal muscles are relatively weaker than distal muscles	0.9	1.2	Muscle grades for proximal muscles in the legs are relatively lower than distal muscles in the legs as defined by manual muscle testing or other objective strength testing
Skin manifestations			
Heliotrope rash	3.1	3.2	Purple, lilac-colored or erythematous patches over the eyelids or in a periorbital distribution, often associated with periorbital edema
Gottron's papules	2.1	2.7	Erythematous to violaceous papules over the extensor surfaces of joints, which are sometimes scaly. May occur over the finger joints, elbows, knees, malleoli, and toes

(continued)

Table 10.7 (continued)

When no better explanation for the symptoms and signs exists, these classification criteria can be used			
Variable	Score points		
	Without muscle biopsy	With muscle biopsy	Definition
Gottron's sign	3.3	3.7	Erythematous to violaceous macules over the extensor surfaces of joints, which are not palpable
Other clinical manifestations			
Dysphagia or esophageal dysmotility	0.7	0.6	Difficulty in swallowing or objective evidence of abnormal motility of the esophagus
Laboratory measurements			
Anti-Jo-1 (anti-histidyl-tRNA synthetase) autoantibody present	3.9	3.8	Autoantibody test in serum performed with standardized and validated test, showing positive result
Elevated serum levels of creatine kinase (CK) *or* lactate dehydrogenase (LDH) *or* aspartate aminotransferase (ASAT/AST/SGOT) *or* alanine aminotransferase (ALAT/ALT/SGPT)	1.3	1.4	The most abnormal test values during the disease course (highest absolute level of enzyme) above the relevant upper limit of normal
Muscle biopsy features: presence of			
Endomysial infiltration of mononuclear cells surrounding, but not invading, myofibers		1.7	Muscle biopsy reveals endomysial mononuclear cells abutting the sarcolemma of otherwise healthy, non-necrotic muscle fibers, but there is no clear invasion of the muscle fibers
Perimysial and/or perivascular infiltration of mononuclear cells		1.2	Mononuclear cells are located in the perimysium and/or located around blood vessels (in either perimysial or endomysial vessels)
Perifascicular atrophy		1.9	Muscle biopsy reveals several rows of muscle fibers which are smaller in the perifascicular region than fibers more centrally located
Rimmed vacuoles		3.1	Rimmed vacuoles are bluish by hematoxylin and eosin staining and reddish by modified Gomori trichrome stains

Adapted from EULAR/ACR Classification Criteria for Adult and Juvenile Idiopathic Inflammatory Myopathies and their Major Subgroups, Ann Rheum Dis. 2018 [10]

10.7 Conclusion

Dermatomyositis is a multifaceted autoimmune condition marked by characteristic cutaneous findings and progressive muscle involvement, often with systemic implications. Its diagnosis relies on a high index of clinical suspicion, especially due to the wide variability in presentation, including amyopathic and hypomyopathic forms. The potential for significant morbidity from systemic involvement and the increased risk of associated malignancies—particularly in adult-onset DM—necessitate a multidisciplinary approach to management.

References

1. Bohan A, Peter JB. Polymyositis and dermatomyositis. N Engl J Med. 1975;292(344–7):403–7.
2. Fornaro M, Girolamo F, Giannini M, Coladonato L, Capuano A, Capodiferro M, d'Abbicco D, Ruggieri M, Mastrapasqua M, Iannone F. Clinical, histologic and prognostic features of clinically amyopathic dermatomyositis. Clin Exp Rheumatol. 2024;42(2)
3. Thompson C, Piguet V, Choy E. The pathogenesis of dermatomyositis. Br J Dermatol. 2018;179(6):1256–62. https://doi.org/10.1111/bjd.15607.
4. Cobos GA, Femia A, Vleugels RA. Dermatomyositis: an update on diagnosis and treatment. Am J Clin Dermatol. 2020;21:339–53. https://doi.org/10.1007/s40257-020-00502-6.
5. Davuluri S, Duvvuri B, Lood C, Faghihi-Kashani S, Chung L. Calcinosis in dermatomyositis: origins and possible therapeutic avenues. Best Pract Res Clin Rheumatol. 2022;36(2):101768. https://doi.org/10.1016/j.berh.2022.101768.
6. Muro Y, Sugiura K, Akiyama M. Cutaneous manifestations in Dermatomyositis: key clinical and serological features – a comprehensive review. Clin Rev Allerg Immunol. 2016;51:293–302. https://doi.org/10.1007/s12016-015-8496-5.
7. Saraya T, Kasuga K, Kishimoto M, Ishii H. Hiker's feet: hidden warning skin sign. Intern Med. 2022;61(16):2551–2. https://doi.org/10.2169/internalmedicine.8999-21.
8. Alfraji N, Mazahir U, Chaudhri M, et al. Anti-synthetase syndrome: a rare and challenging diagnosis for bilateral ground-glass opacities – a case report with literature review. BMC Pulm Med. 2021;21:11. https://doi.org/10.1186/s12890-020-01388-0.
9. Bogdanov I, Kazandjieva J, Darlenski R, Tsankov N. Dermatomyositis: current concepts. Clin Dermatol. 2018;36(4):450–8.
10. Lundberg IE, Tjärnlund A, Bottai M, Werth VP, Pilkington C, Visser M, et al. Ann Rheum Dis. 2017;76(12):1955–64.

Sjogren's Syndrome

11

Sapan Pandya and Kunal Chandwar

Abstract

Sjogren's syndrome is known to be the commonest autoimmune rheumatic illness. Classically a B cell-mediated disease with type I interferon signatures in the majority of cases, the role of cholinergic system especially muscarinic receptors also is coming into focus. Predominantly manifested as dry mouth and dry eyes, it has a range of extraglandular manifestations like renal tubular acidosis, demyelinating illness, and purpura which present more to the rheumatologist as a referral bias. The importance of therapy is because of its likelihood to evolve into a lymphoma in a subset of cases. While the usual investigations like Schirmer's test, lissamine green test for dry eye, salivary flow rates for dry mouth, and autoantibodies are done, salivary ultrasound is coming to replace biopsies in recent times. The latest classification criteria have a scoring system for clinical trials. Therapy is still largely the same with topical ointments for sicca, pilocarpine for dry mouth, and immunosuppressive drugs for the more aggressive ones—ianalumab seems a promising new biologic. Prognosis is now better with earlier diagnosis and treatment.

Keywords

Sjogren's syndrome · Sicca · Purpura

S. Pandya (✉)
Department of Rheumatology, SVPIMSR, Smt NHL Municipal Medical College, Ahmedabad, India

K. Chandwar
Department of Clinical Immunology and Rheumatology, Sanjay Gandhi Postgraduate Institute of Medical Sciences, Lucknow, India

P. Agarwal et al. (eds.), *Dermatologist's Handbook of Autoimmune Connective Tissue Diseases*, https://doi.org/10.1007/978-981-95-0524-1_11

11.1 Introduction

Sjögren's syndrome (SS) is a systemic autoimmune exocrinopathy leading to dryness of the main mucosal surfaces—the mouth, eyes, skin, nose, pharynx, larynx, and vagina. The clinical spectrum of SS extends from dryness of the main mucosal surfaces to systemic involvement (extraglandular manifestations), leading to wide-ranging manifestations. The variability in the presentation often leads to delays in diagnosis (up to 10 years from the onset of symptoms).

- Primary Sjögren's syndrome (pSS): When the syndrome is not associated with another immune-mediated inflammatory disorder (IMID).
- Secondary Sjögren's syndrome (sSS): When there is overlap with another IMID.

11.2 Etiopathogenesis

The etiopathogenesis is explained in Fig. 11.1.

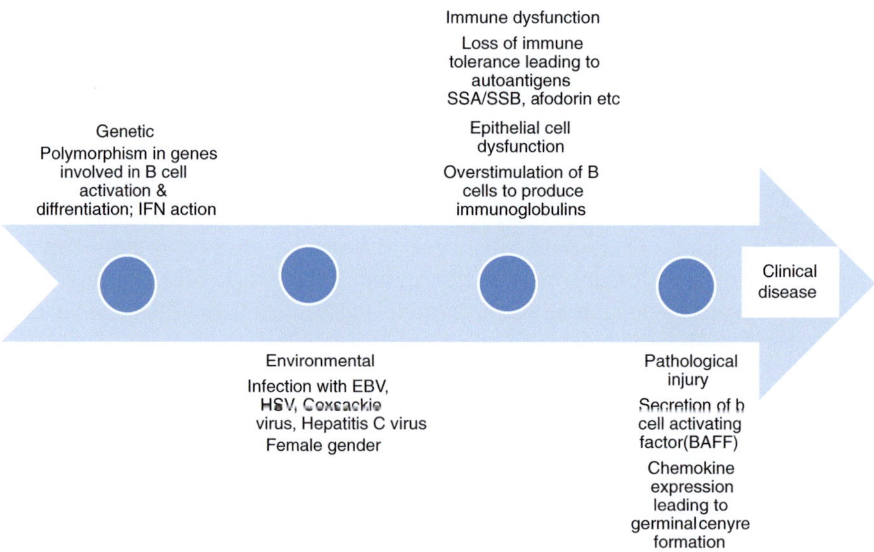

Fig. 11.1 Etiopathogenesis of Sjögren's syndrome

11.3 Clinical Features [1, 2]

A dermatologist should suspect a possibility of Sjögren's syndrome when a patient presents with:

- Purpura over lower limbs which increases on dangling the legs and decreases in supine position (hypergammaglobulinemic purpura).
- Annular erythema.
- Excessive dry skin with dryness of mouth and eyes.
- Panniculitis lesions associated with sicca symptoms.
- Urticaria associated with sicca symptoms.
- Parotid or submandibular swelling (Fig. 11.2).
- Peripheral neuropathy (after exclusion of other causes).
- In mother of a child born with congenital heart block.

Once suspected, it is important to look for signs and symptoms suggestive of systemic involvement. The patient may also have chronic fatigue and fibromyalgia like symptoms. The plethora of systemic manifestations is mentioned in Tables 11.1 and Fig. 11.3.

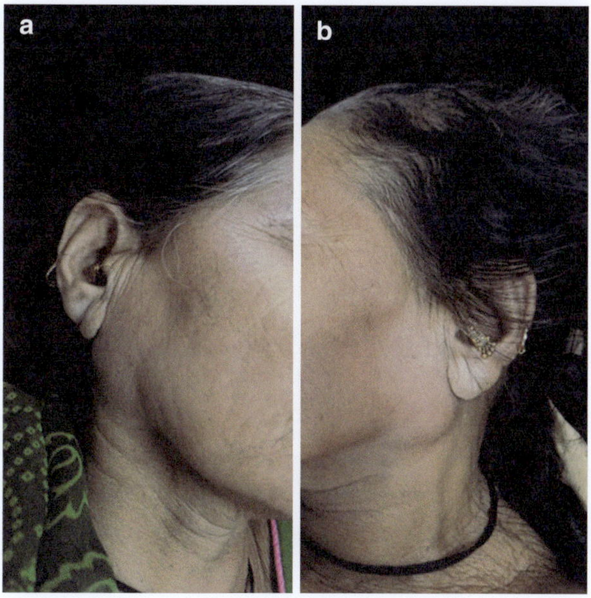

Fig. 11.2 (**a**, **b**) Bilateral parotid gland swelling

Table 11.1 Sicca signs and symptoms suggestive of Sjögren's syndrome

Oral	Ocular	Others
Soreness	Photosensitivity	Persistent hoarseness
Adherence of food to the mucosa	Erythema	Pruritus in the outer ear and ear canal
Dysphagia	Eye fatigue	Chronic, nonproductive cough
Difficulties in speaking or eating	Decreased visual acuity	Cutaneous dryness
Tooth decay	Blepharitis	Dyspareunia
Periodontal disease	Bacterial keratitis	Vaginal pruritus
Difficulty with dentures	Conjunctivitis	
Disappearance of the usual pooling of saliva in the floor of the mouth	Corneal ulceration	
Surface of the tongue red and lobulated	Corneal vascularization and opacification	
Partial or complete depapillation of the tongue		
Dry and glazed oral mucosa		
Fine wrinkles in the oral mucosa		
Angular cheilitis		
Erythematous changes of the hard palate		
Red tongue with atrophic papillae		
Candida infection		

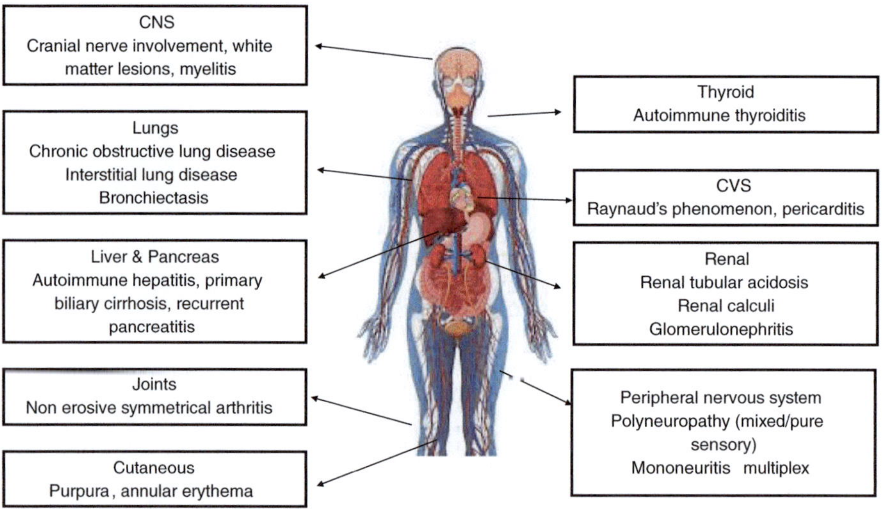

Fig. 11.3 Major systemic/extraglandular manifestations of Sjögren's syndrome [3]

11.4 Classification Criteria for Sjogren's Syndrome

- Several classification criteria for Sjögren's syndrome have been published since the 1960s.
- 2002 American European Consensus group (AECG) [4] and the 2016 ACR-EULAR [5] criteria have been the most widely (Table 11.2).

Table 11.2 Comparison of American European Consensus Group (AECG) and EULAR/ACR Criteria for the classification of primary Sjögren syndrome

2002 American European Consensus Group (AECG)	EULAR/ACR criteria	Score
Inclusion criteria		
Ocular dryness symptoms	Labial salivary gland with focal lymphocytic sialadenitis and a focus score of ≥1 (A focus score is the number of inflammatory infiltrates of at least 50 cells present in 4 mm^2 of gland surface unit)	3
Oral dryness symptom	Anti-SSA antibodies (anti-Ro)	3
Ocular signs: Schirmer's test ≤5 mm/5 min or van Bijsterveld score ≥4	Ocular staining score ≥5 (or van Bijsterveld score ≥4) in at least 1 eye	1
Focus score ≥1 foci/4 mm^2 on minor salivary gland biopsy	Schirmer's test ≤5 mm/5 min in at least 1 eye [6]	1
Salivary gland involvement: unstimulated whole salivary flow ≤0.1 mL/min	Unstimulated whole saliva flow rate ≤0.1 mL/min [7]	1
Positive anti-SSA or SSB antibodies	–	–
Common to both classification: History of radiation treatment to the head and neck, active hepatitis C infection (confirmed by polymerase chain reaction), advanced HIV infection, sarcoidosis, amyloidosis, graft-vs-host disease, IgG4-related disease *Additional in AECG:* Pre-existing lymphoma, use of anticholinergic drugs (within a time shorter than fourfold the half-life of the drug) *Additional in EULAR/ACR:* Amyloidosis, IgG4-related disease		
1. Presence of any 4 of the 6 items with at least item 4 or 6 2. Presence of any 3 of the 4 objective items (3, 4, 5, and 6)	A score ≥4 classifies a patient who meets the inclusion criteria Ocular and/or oral dryness or suspicion of SjS according to EULAR SjSA disease activity index (ESSDAI)	

11.5 Differential Diagnosis [8, 9]

A number of diseases may mimic Sjögren's syndrome, and it is necessary to maintain a high degree of suspicion (Table 11.3).

Table 11.3 Diseases mimicking Sjögren's syndrome

	Signs/symptoms mimicking Sjogren's	Differentiation from Sjogren's
Diabetes mellitus	Sicca	Usually diagnosed cases; blood sugars
Sarcoidosis	Sicca/parotitis/peripheral neuropathy	Biopsy, absence of autoantibodies (ANAs)
Tuberculosis	Parotitis/submandibular gland enlargement	Biopsy, absence of autoantibodies (ANAs)
HCV	Sicca/cryoglobulins	HCV status, absence of ANAs
HIV	Sicca/parotitis	Biopsy, HIV status, absence of anti Ro/La
Amyloidosis	Sicca/rashes/raised globulins in blood	Biopsy/serum electrophoresis/absence of ANAs
IgG4-related disease	Parotitis/lacrimal gland involvement	Biopsy/absence of ANAs
Lymphoma	Parotitis/submandibular gland enlargement/cryoglobulins	Biopsy with immunohistochemistry
Drugs like anti-histaminics/anti-depressants	Sicca	History of the drug's usage/absence of ANAs
Ocular rosacea	Xerophthalmia	Absence of ANAs
Chronic GVHD	Xerophthalmia; xerostomia	History of transplant; absence of ANAs

11.6 Conclusion

Suspect Sjogren's syndrome in patients presenting with dry skin with dry mouth and/or eyes (much more commonly seen with conditions like diabetes but one should ask questions about SS clinical features and get an ANA by IIF done if you suspect).

Those with hypergammaglobulinemic purpura (recurrent purpura lower limbs increasing in dependent position) or palpable purpura with Raynaud's/inflammatory joint pains and/or parotitis warrant investigations for SS.

References

1. Kittridge A, Routhouska SB, Korman NJ. Dermatologic manifestations of Sjögren syndrome. J Cutan Med Surg. 2011;15:14–8.
2. De Oliveira FR, Fantucci MZ, Adriano L, Valim V, Cunha TM, Louzada-Junior P, Rocha EM. Neurological and inflammatory manifestations in Sjögren's syndrome: the role of the kynurenine metabolic pathway. Int J Mol Sci. 2018;19(12):3953. https://doi.org/10.3390/ijms19123953.
3. Ramos-Casals M, Brito-Zerón P, Sisó-Almirall A, Bosch X. Primary Sjogren syndrome. BMJ. 2012;344:e3821. https://doi.org/10.1136/bmj.e3821.
4. Vitali C, Bombardieri S, Jonsson R, Moutsopoulos HM, Alexander EL, Carsons SE, et al. Classification criteria for Sjogren's syndrome: a revised version of the European criteria proposed by the American-European Consensus Group. Ann Rheum Dis. 2002;61:554–8.
5. Le Goff M, Cornec D, Jousse-Joulin S, Guellec D, Costa S, Marhadour T, Le Berre R, Genestet S, Cochener B, Boisrame-Gastrin S, Renaudineau Y, Pers JO, Saraux A, Devauchelle-Pensec V. Comparison of 2002 AECG and 2016 ACR/EULAR classification criteria and added value of salivary gland ultrasonography in a patient cohort with suspected primary Sjögren's syndrome. Arthritis Res Ther. 2017;19(1):269. https://doi.org/10.1186/s13075-017-1475-x. PMID: 29208023; PMCID: PMC5717850.
6. A simplified quantitative method for assessing keratoconjunctivitis sicca from the Sjögren's syndrome international registry. Am J Ophthalmol. 2010;149(3):405–15. https://doi.org/10.1016/j.ajo.2009.09.013.
7. Methods for collecting saliva. Ann NY Acad Sci. 1993;694:72–7. https://doi.org/10.1111/j.1749-6632.1993.tb18343.x.
8. Mavragani CP, Moutsopoulos HM. Sjögren syndrome. CMAJ. 2014;186(15):E579–86. https://doi.org/10.1503/cmaj.122037. Epub 2014 Feb 24. PMID: 24566651; PMCID: PMC4203623.
9. Carsons SE, Patel BC. Sjogren syndrome. [Updated 2023 July 31]. In: StatPearls [Internet]. Treasure Island (FL): StatPearls Publishing; 2025 Jan-. Available from: https://www.ncbi.nlm.nih.gov/books/NBK431049/

Mixed Connective Tissue Disease, Overlap, and Undifferentiated Connective Tissue Disease

12

Puja Srivastava

Abstract

At the onset, many autoimmune connective tissue diseases (CTDs) are not fully evolved, and this early stage of the disease is known as undifferentiated connective tissue disease (UCTD). Approximately, 50% of cases of UCTDs remain undifferentiated throughout the disease course. All major CTDs have varying degrees of overlap in clinical features, and the degree of overlap correlates with their genetic and autoantibody profiles. Mixed connective tissue disease (MCTD) is a distinct prototype overlap syndrome with clinical features from lupus, rheumatoid arthritis, scleroderma, and myositis. Raynaud's phenomenon is the most common presentation among patients with UCTD, overlap CTDs, and MCTD.

Keywords

Raynaud's phenomenon · UCTD · MCTD · Overlap syndrome · ANA · Nailfold capillaroscopy

12.1 Introduction

- Many patients with CTD do not develop all the classical clinical features of the disease at onset, rather they add new symptoms and signs as the disease evolves over time. Thus, in the early stage, these autoimmune CTDs may not be well differentiated, and this stage of their evolution is called "undifferentiated connective tissue disease (UCTD)" [1].

P. Srivastava (✉)
Department of Immunology & Rheumatology, STAR Clinics, Ahmedabad, India

P. Agarwal et al. (eds.), *Dermatologist's Handbook of Autoimmune Connective Tissue Diseases*, https://doi.org/10.1007/978-981-95-0524-1_12

Table 12.1 Nomenclature for connective tissue diseases (CTDs)

Undifferentiated connective tissue disease	Does not fulfill criteria of any given CTD, but has early features suggestive of an autoimmune disease (may progress to a particular path in the future)
Overlap syndrome	Patients fulfill classification criteria of at least two different CTD simultaneously or at different occasion
Mixed connective tissue disease	Well-defined CTD, with very high ANA titers and U1-RNP-positive status

- Many patients, with early undifferentiated CTD, evolve into one of the well-defined classic CTDs over time. The propensity for maintenance of UCTD phenotype or differentiation into classic CTD depends on distinctive autoantibody profile and genetic major histocompatibility (MHC) linkages [2].
- Although rare, sometimes it has been observed that over years, one established CTD may change phenotype to evolve into another CTD.
- Mixed connective-tissue disease (MCTD) is an overlap syndrome with clinical features of lupus, systemic sclerosis, rheumatoid arthritis, and inflammatory myositis. It was first recognized as a distinct entity in 1972 by Sharp and colleagues [3]. It was also the first overlap syndrome characterized by a specific autoantibody against U1-ribonucleoprotein (U1-RNP) along with very high titers (often >1:1000) of anti-nuclear antibody (ANA) positivity [4]. Over years there have been multiple efforts to create a standardized diagnostic criterion for MCTD.
- Nomenclature of CTDs are listed in Table 12.1, It is important to note that a patient with UCTD can evolve intoany of the six well defined CTDs in future.

12.2 Pathogenesis

Autoimmunity and Vasculopathy [5–9].

- The anti-U1-RNP antibody and its antigen are believed to play a crucial role in the pathogenesis of mixed connective tissue disease. The U1-RNP complex in the nucleus has three specific proteins—A, C, and 70 kDa. The anti-U1 RNP antibodies bind to these antigens with the 70 kDa antigen being the main target in MCTD.
- There is a genetic association with HLA—B*08 and DRB1*04:01 phenotypes which indicate the role of T cell receptors in the formation of anti-U1-RNP antibodies. HLA DRB1*04:04, DRB1*13:01, and DRB1*13:02 are protective against MCTD.
- The two main proposed mechanisms for the pathogenic role of anti-U1-RNP antibodies are shown in Fig. 12.1.

The summation of pathophysiologic abnormalities which are believed to play a role in MCTD is explained in Fig. 12.2.

Fig. 12.1 Proposed pathogenic mechanism for anti-U1-RNP antibodies

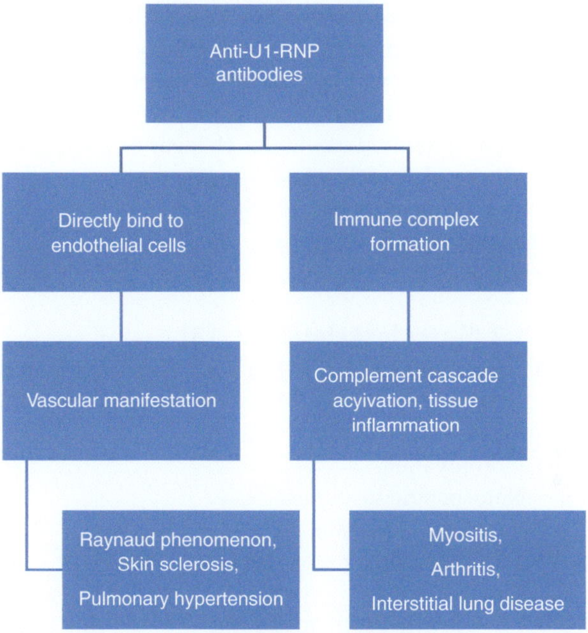

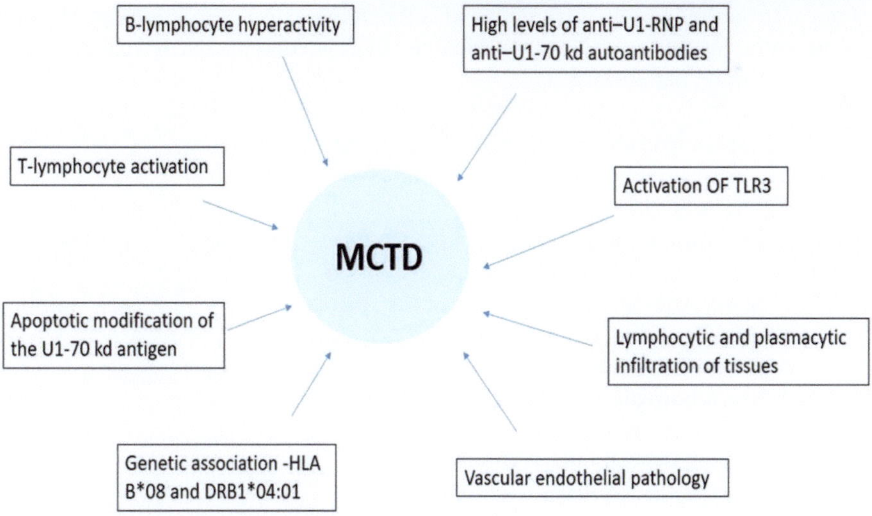

Fig. 12.2 Pathogenesis of MCTD

12.3 MCTD

12.3.1 Clinical Features

MCTD is the prototype overlap syndrome, characterized by clinical features of different well-defined CTDs [10].

12.3.1.1 Mucocutaneous Manifestations of MCTD/UCTD [11]

- Raynaud's phenomenon is usually the earliest symptom, and there is an accompanying puffy swelling of hands and feet, may ocasionally cause sausage-shaped swelling of the digits.
- Prominent nailfold capillaries changes or periungual telangiectasia.
- Small vessel vasculitis and palpable purpura.
- Erythematous plaques resembling discoid lupus erythematosus.
- Facial erythema.
- Sclerosis of the skin.

12.3.1.2 Musculoskeletal [12, 13]

- Malaise, myositis, and arthritis are among the common noncutaneous features.
- Arthralgia and arthritis: More severe arthritis as compared to lupus.
- Muscle involvement.
  - Fibromyalgia.
  - Non-specific myalgias.
  - Subclinical myositis.
  - Frank inflammatory myositis.

12.3.1.3 Cardio-Pulmonary Manifestations [14, 15]

- Pulmonary artery hypertension (PAH): the most common and most severe form of cardio-pulmonary involvement and is the major cause of mortality in MCTD.
- Interstitial lung disease: Non-specific interstitial pneumonia (NSIP) pattern is the most common pattern of ILD.

12.3.1.4 Gastrointestinal (GI) Manifestations [16, 17]

- Esophageal dysmotility: dyspepsia and reflux symptoms can progress to esophageal strictures and cancer.
- Lower GI hypomotility: constipation can progress to small intestinal bacterial overgrowth syndrome (SIBO) and malabsorption.
- Others manifestation: ascites, pancreatitis, primary biliary cirrhosis, autoimmune hepatitis, and mesenteric vasculitis.

12.3.1.5 Hematological Involvement [18]

- Autoimmune hemolytic anemia (AIHA).
- Positive Coombs test in up to 60% cases.
- Leukopenia: marker of disease activity.
- Thrombocytopenia.
- Positive lupus anticoagulant and anti-cardiolipin antibodies associate with vasculopathy and increased mortality.

12.3.1.6 Nervous System Manifestations (Rare) [18, 19]

- Trigeminal neuralgia (TN) is the commonest presentation.
- Cognitive dysfunction, convulsions, and psychosis are rare as compared to lupus.

On magnetic resonance imaging (MRI): unspecific bright objects (UBOs) may be seen in different areas of the brain, this may or may not correlate with the clinical manifestation.

12.3.1.7 Renal Manifestations (Rare) [20]

- Mild and asymptomatic.
- Membranous glomerulonephritis is commonest form of glomerular pathology in this disease.
- Presence of anti-U1-RNP antibody: protective against the development of diffuse proliferative glomerulonephritis.
- Increased risk of scleroderma like renal crisis (especially after prolonged high dose corticosteroids therapy).

12.3.2 Classification Criteria

Over the years, there have been various efforts to create a standardized diagnostic criterion for MCTD. The four criteria that have stood the test of time are the Sharp's criteria, the Kasukawa diagnostic criteria, the Alarcón-Segovia criteria, and the Kahn criteria. Although comparisons among the criteria are limited, the Alarcón-Segovia and Kahn criteria have demonstrated the best sensitivity and specificity (Table 12.2) [21], while the Kasukawa criteria have the best sensitivity.

Hence, the former two criteria should be used to "rule in" a disease, while the latter should be used to "rule out" the disease.

Table 12.2 Various diagnostic criteria for MCTD

Name	Diagnostic criteria	
Sharp	**Major criteria**	**Minor criteria**
At least 4 major criteria plus anti-U1-RNP antibody titer of at least 1:1000 **or** Two major criteria from among criteria 1, 2, and 3 **plus** 2 minor criteria **plus** anti-U1-RNP Antibody titer of at least 1:1000 **Exclusion criteria**: Positivity for anti-Sm Ab	1. Myositis 2. Pulmonary involvement: Diffusion capacity <70% of normal values Pulmonary hypertension Proliferative vascular lesions on lung biopsy 3. Raynaud's phenomenon oresophageal hypomotility 4. Swollen hands 5. Anti-ENA Ab N 1:10,000 and anti-U1-RNP Ab positive and anti-Sm negative	1. Alopecia 2. Leukopenia 3. Anemia 4. Pleuritis 5. Pericarditis 6. Arthritis 7. Trigeminal neuropathy 8. Malar rash 9. Thrombocytopenia 10. Mild myositis 11. History of swollen hands

(continued)

Table 12.2 (continued)

Name	Diagnostic criteria	
Kasukawa	**Common symptoms**	**Mixed symptoms**
At least one of common symptoms **plus** positivity for anti-RNP Antibody **plus** one or more signs/ symptoms of the mixed symptoms in at least two of the three disease categories	1. Raynaud's phenomenon 2. Swollen fingers or hands anti-RNP Ab positive	1. SLE-like symptoms: Polyarthritis Lymphadenopathy Facial erythema Pericarditis or pleuritis Leukopenia or thrombocytopenia 2. SSc-like findings: Sclerodactyly Pulmonary fibrosis, restrictive changes of lung, or reduced diffusion capacity Hypomotility or dilatation of the esophagus 3. PM-like findings: Muscle weakness Elevated serum levels of muscle enzymes (CPK) Myogenic pattern on EMG
Alarcón-Segovi	**Serological criteria**	**Clinical criteria**
Serological criteria plus at least three clinical criteria included either synovitis or myositis	Anti-RNP Ab titer N 1:1000	1. Edema in hands 2. synovitis 3. myositis 4. Raynaud's phenomenon 5. Acrosclerosis
Kahn	**Serological criteria**	**Clinical criteria**
Serological criteria plus Raynaud's phenomenon and at least two of the three following signs Synovitis Myositis Swollen fingers	Presence of high titer anti-RNP Ab corresponding to speckled ANA at titer ≥1:2000	1. Raynaud's phenomenon 2. Synovitis 3. Myositis 4. Swollen fingers

12.4 Overlap Syndromes

12.4.1 Scleroderma Overlap Syndromes [22–24]

Systemic sclerosis often overlaps with different CTDs, and in few epidemiological studies, overlap disease has been found to be more common than the primary form of the disease.

- More common in patients without skin involvement (sine scleroderma) or in those with limited forms of the disease like CREST.
- The patients with overlap disease have specific antibody associations and mostly have good long-term prognosis.

- CREST syndrome is frequently associated with overlap features with Sjogren's syndrome (SS), primary biliary cirrhosis (PBC), and rheumatoid arthritis.

Anti-mitochondrial antibodies (AMA) have shown to be associated with PBC and limited forms of SSc.

- Polymyositis-scleroderma overlap: Anti PM-Scl antibodies are most commonly associated with polymyositis-scleroderma overlap. Despite higher pulmonary and muscle involvement, this subgroup of patients have better survival as compared to patients with diffuse SSc. Presence of Ku antibody is also associated with overlap myositis in SSc patients.

12.4.2 Lupus Overlap Syndromes [25, 26]

As compared to SSc, overlap syndromes are less common in SLE.

1. An overlap of lupus and Sjogren's syndrome (SS) occurs in about 10–25% patients, and presence of anti-SS-A and SS-B antibodies at the time of diagnosis predicts higher likelihood of eventual development of SLE-SS overlap. Patients with this overlap syndrome have higher frequency of Raynaud's syndrome and lower frequency of thrombocytopenia, lymphadenopathy, and renal involvement.
2. RA and SLE overlap has been seen in ~10% of SLE patients and is commonly referred as "Rhupus." The typical clinical picture is the presence of erosive and deforming polyarthritis in a patient with clinical picture of SLE. They are often associated with high titers of rheumatoid factor (RF) and anti-CCP antibodies. Patients with rhupus often have less severe renal involvement.

12.4.3 Myositis Overlap Syndromes [22, 27]

Overlap syndromes of inflammatory myositis with SSc, SLE, and SS and RA are quite common.

- These overlaps are more common than primary PM/DM phenotypes and have better long-term prognosis.
- Apart from prognostic role, autoantibody profile of overlap myositis also has therapeutic significance, where presence of anti-SRP, anti-nucleoporin, and anti-synthetase antibodies is an associated refractory disease.
- Patients with dermatomyositis (primary and overlap syndromes) are associated with increased risk of malignancy.

12.5 Conclusions

Most patients with CTDs are ill-defined at presentation, and they evolve over time from undifferentiated syndromes into either well-defined distinct CTDs or into different overlap syndromes. Autoantibody profiles provide some idea as to which way the patients with UCTD/overlap syndromes are likely to evolve over the years. MCTD is the prototype overlap syndrome, with distinct autoantibody profile and classification criteria. In general, most UCTDs, overlap syndromes, and MCTD have a better long-term outcome and survival, when compared to well-defined distinct CTDs like lupus.

References

1. LeRoy EC, Maricq H, Kahaleh M. Undifferentiated connective tissue syndrome. Arthritis Rheum. 1980;23:341–3.
2. Bodolay E, Csiki Z, Szekanecz Z, et al. Five year follow up of 665 Hungarian patients with undifferentiated connective tissue disease (UCTD). Clin Exp Rheumatol. 2003;21(3):313–20.
3. Sharp GC, Irvin WS, Tan EM, et al. Mixed connective tissue disease—an apparently distinct rheumatic disease syndrome associated with a specific antibody to an extractable nuclear antigen (ENA). Am J Med. 1972;52(2):148–59.
4. Tanaka Y, Kuwana M, Fujii T, Kameda H, Muro Y, Fujio K, et al. 2019 diagnostic criteria for mixed connective tissue disease (MCTD): from the Japan research committee of the ministry of health, labour, and welfare for systemic autoimmune diseases. Mod Rheumatol. 2021;31:29–33.
5. Paradowska-Gorycka A. U1-RNP and TLR receptors in the pathogenesis of mixed connective tissue disease. Part I. The U1-RNP complex and its biological significance in the pathogenesis of mixed connective tissue disease. Reumatologia. 2015;53(2):94–100. https://doi.org/10.5114/reum.2015.51509. Epub 2015 May 18. PMID: 27407234; PMCID: PMC4847272.
6. Hoffman RW, Rettenmaier LJ, Takeda Y, et al. Human autoantibodies against the 70-kd polypeptide of U1 small nuclear RNP are associated with HLA-DR4 among connective tissue disease patients. Arthritis Rheum. 1990;33(5):666–73. https://doi.org/10.1002/art.1780330509.
7. Paradowska-Gorycka A, Wajda A, Stypinska B, Walczuk E, Rzeszotarska E, Walczyk M, et al. Variety of endosomal TLRs and interferons (IFN-α, IFN-β, IFN-γ) expression profiles in patients with SLE, SSc and MCTD. Clin Exp Immunol. 2020; https://doi.org/10.1111/cei.13566.
8. Escolà-Vergé L, Pinal-Fernandez I, Fernandez-Codina A, Callejas-Moraga EL, Espinosa J, Marin A, et al. Mixed connective tissue disease and epitope spreading: an historical cohort study. J Clin Rheumatol. 2017;23(3):155–9.
9. Flåm ST, Gunnarsson R, Garen T, Norwegian MCTD Study Group, Lie BA, Molberg Ø. The HLA profiles of mixed connective tissue disease differ distinctly from the profiles of clinically related connective tissue diseases. Rheumatology (Oxford). 2015;54(3):528–35.
10. Bennet RM. Overlap syndromes. In: Kelly's and Firestein textbook of rheumatology, vol. 2. Philadelphia: Elsevier; 2017. p. 1489–511.
11. Cansu DÜ, Korkmaz C. Pulmonary hypertension in connective tissue diseases: epidemiology, pathogenesis, and treatment. Clin Rheumatol. 2023;42(10):2601–10.
12. Szodoray P, Hazas A, Kardos L, et al. Distinct phenotypes in mixed connective tissue disease: subgroups and survival. Lupus. 2012;21(13):1412–22.
13. Vianna MA, Borges CT, Borba EF, et al. Myositis in MCTD a unique syndrome characterised by immunohistopathologic elements of polymyositis and dermatomyositis. Arq Neuropsiquiatr. 2004;62(4):923–34.

14. Ungprasert P, Wannarong T, Panichsillapakit T, et al. Cardiac involvement in mixed connective tissue disease (MCTD): a systematic review. Int J Cardiol. 2014;171(3):326–30.
15. Hant FN, Herpel LB, Silver RM. Pulmonary manifestations of scleroderma and mixed connective tissue disease (MCTD). Clin Chest Med. 2010;31(3):433–49.
16. Pope JE. Other manifestations of mixed connective tissue disease. Rheum Dis Clin N Am. 2005;31(3):519–33.
17. Uzuki M, Kamataki A, Watanabe M, et al. Histological analysis of esophageal muscular layers from 27 autopsy cases with mixed connective tissue disease (MCTD). Pathol Res Pract. 2011;207(6):383–90.
18. Hazas A, Szodoray P, Nakken B, et al. Clinical course, prognosis and causes of death in mixed connective tissue disease. J Rheumatol. 2013;40(7):1134–42.
19. Hajas A, Szodoray P, Barath S, et al. Sensorineural hearing loss in patients with mixed connective tissue disease: immunological markers and cytokine levels. J Rheumatol. 2009;39(9):930–6.
20. Kitridou RC, Akmal M, Turkel SB, et al. Renal involvement in mixed connective tissue disease: a longitudinal clinicopathologic study. Semin Arthritis Rheum. 1986;16(2):135–45.
21. John KJ, Sadiq M, George T, Gunasekaran K, Francis N, Rajadurai E, Sudarsanam TD. Clinical and immunological profile of mixed connective tissue disease and a comparison of four diagnostic criteria. Int J Rheumatol. 2020;2020(1):9692030.
22. Troyanov Y, Targoff IN, Tremblay JL, et al. Novel classification of idiopathic inflammatory myopathies based on overlap syndrome features and autoantibodies: analysis of 100 French Canadian patients. Medicine (Baltimore). 2005;84(4):231–49.
23. Miyawaki S, Asanuma H, Nishiyama S, et al. Clinical and serological heterogeneity in patients with anticentromere antibodies. J Rheumatol. 2005;32(8):1488–94.
24. Koschik RW, Fertig N, Lucas MR, et al. Anti-PM-Scl antibody in patients with systemic sclerosis. Clin Exp Rheumatol. 2012;30(2 Suppl 71):s12–6.
25. Manoussakis MN, Georgopoulou C, Zintzaras E, et al. Sjogren's syndrome associated with systemic lupus erythematosus: clinical and laboratory profiles and comparison with primary Sjogrens syndrome. Arthritis Rheum. 2004;50(3):882–91.
26. Tani C, D'Aniello D, Delle SA, et al. Rhupus syndrome: assessment of its prevalence and its clinical and instrumental characteristics in a prospective cohort of 103 SLE patients. Autoimmun Rev. 2013;12(4):537–41.
27. Chen YJ, Wu CY, Huang YL, et al. Cancer risks of dermatomyositis and polymyositis: a nationwide cohort study in Taiwan. Arthritis Res Ther. 2010;12(2):R20.

Part III

Management of the CTDs

Management of Raynaud's Phenomenon 13

Ankan Gupta and Kriteeka Saini

Abstract

The overall goal in the management of Raynaud's is to decrease the intensity and severity of attacks and improve the quality of life. Primary Raynaud's is generally a benign condition which can be managed with non-pharmacological interventions alone in most cases, whereas pharmacotherapy is generally required in most cases of secondary Raynaud's. Long-acting calcium channel blockers such as amlodipine or nifedipine are the drugs of choice. Other classes of drugs include phosphodiesterase-5 inhibitors, prostacyclin analogs, topical nitrates, etc. Surgical interventions are generally reserved for severe and unresponsive cases.

Keywords

Raynaud's · Calcium channel blockers · Iloprost · Bosentan · Phosphodiesterase-5 inhibitors

13.1 Introduction

Raynaud's phenomenon is characterized by transient digital ischemia in response to cold temperature or emotional distress. It is caused by vasoconstriction of the digital arteries, precapillary arterioles, and cutaneous arteriovenous shunts [1].

Patient education and avoidance of triggers form the cornerstone of management in both primary and secondary Raynaud's phenomenon. Unresponsive cases are

A. Gupta
Department of Dermatology, Blacktown Dermatology, Sydney, NSW, Australia

K. Saini (✉)
Kavach Skin Clinic, Mhow, Madhya Pradesh, India

P. Agarwal et al. (eds.), *Dermatologist's Handbook of Autoimmune Connective Tissue Diseases*, https://doi.org/10.1007/978-981-95-0524-1_13

subsequently initiated on pharmacotherapy or surgical procedures like sympathectomy [2].

All management strategies are aimed to decrease the intensity and frequency of symptoms, prevent visible anatomical disfiguration of fingers, and maintain the dexterity or daily functioning of fingers. Abolishing cold sensitivity and eliminating all Raynaud events are not likely with the available treatment options.

13.2 Non-pharmacological Interventions

13.2.1 Patient Education and Avoidance Strategies [2–4]

- All patients of Raynaud's phenomenon should be counselled in detail about recognizing the potential triggers and avoiding them to prevent an episode. Even a brief exposure to cold such as placing the hand inside the refrigerator or freezer or using a mixer/grinder or any vibratory tool can precipitate an attack, if overlooked by the patient.
- An important recommendation is to keep the entire body warm and not limit the cold protection to only the acral areas. This can be achieved by using multiple layers of warm clothing and use of indoor heating equipment.
- Emphasize the importance of smoking cessation and limiting caffeine intake.
- Counselling about avoiding anxiety and emotional stress and encouraging behavioral techniques for stress management.
- Avoiding sympathomimetic drugs such as decongestants, amphetamines, and methylphenidate and substituting them for a different class of drug.

13.2.2 Aborting the Attack

Common methods of rewarming acral areas such as rubbing hands against each other, blowing into a closed fist, placing hands in the axillae, or rubbing them with clothing, during an episode of RP, are an integral part of general advice.

13.3 Pharmacotherapy [3–6]

Drug therapy is initiated in patients with primary Raynaud's not responding to non-pharmacological measures alone and in most cases of secondary Raynaud's.

13.3.1 Calcium Channel Blockers

Long-acting dihydropyridine calcium channel blockers (CCB) like nifedipine or amlodipine are the treatment of choice. They are started at the lowest dose and gradually titrated four weekly based on the response, up to the least required dose.

In case of suboptimal response or unacceptable intolerance to therapy, another CCB such as nicardipine, nimodipine, or isradipine may be used.

- Dosage: Amlodipine, 5–20 mg/day; nifedipine 30–180 mg/day.
- Duration of therapy: Not defined, depends on the severity of the episode and underlying cause and sometimes can be indefinite. Individual episode may take up to 6–8 weeks of continuous treatment.
- Cautions: Monitor blood pressure, gastrointestinal dysmotility, significant cardiac disease.
- Adverse effects: Hypotension, peripheral edema, headache, flushing, palpitations, reflex tachycardia, and dose-related dizziness.

13.3.2 Phosphodiesterase Type 5 Inhibitors (PDE-5i)

Alternative therapies such as PDE-5i may be required in patients where CCB are contraindicated or poorly tolerated. PDE-5i may be the drug of choice in patients with secondary Raynaud's with concomitant pulmonary hypertension.

- Dosage: Sildenafil 25–100 mg; tadalafil 5–20 mg.
- Duration of therapy: Not defined, can be indefinite. Mean time of ulcer healing can be about 5 weeks, and fingertip necrosis may take up to 8 weeks for resolution.
- Cautions: Monitor blood pressure.
- Adverse effects: Hypotension, peripheral edema, palpitations, and blue-green visual tinge.

13.3.3 Prostanoid Therapy

Prostacyclin analogs such as iloprost and epoprostenol are administered intravenously in cases of refractory digital ulcers to foster ulcer healing and reduce new ulceration. They are used in patients with severe RP with tissue ischemia or threatened limb loss.

13.3.4 Endothelin Antagonists

Bosentan, an endothelin-1 receptor antagonist, can be used in the management of recurrent digit ulceration seen in connective tissue disorders. Bosentan reduces the development of new ulcers but does not impact on the healing of existing ulcers.

13.3.5 Topical Nitrates

Topical nitrates can induce local direct vasodilatation and may be tried in resistant cases. Typically, a 2% nitroglycerine ointment is applied to the affected areas.

Topical nitrates are absorbed systemically and may result in adverse effects, such as hypotension, dizziness, and headache. *Topical nitrates should not be used together with PDE 5i due to the increased risk of hypotension.*

13.3.6 Anti-platelet and Anticoagulant Drugs

Anti-platelet therapy with low-dose aspirin is generally recommended in the setting of secondary RP with a history of ischemic ulceration caused by structural vessel damage. In the case of intolerance or contraindication to aspirin, clopidogrel or dipyridamole may be used.

Anticoagulant therapy may be considered during the acute phase of digital ischemia in patients with suspected vascular occlusive disease attributed to the occurrence of new thromboses [7].

Other treatment options include angiotensin receptor blocker (ARB) and serotonin reuptake inhibitor (SSRI).

- ARBs are generally chosen as a renoprotective agent in connective tissue disease and for prevention for proteinuria and may help in Raynaud's phenomenon also.
- SSRIs are generally used in combination with first-line agents owing to a different adverse effect profile [8, 9].

There are many trials on the use of pentoxifylline, zinc, N-acetylcysteine, and other antioxidant therapies; however there is limited data to support their use [1, 10, 11].

13.4 Surgical Therapy

Before resorting to procedural therapy, avoidance strategies must be re-emphasized, and compliance to pharmacotherapy must be ensured. Surgical therapy is reserved for severe RP often with persistent digital ischemia.

Indications

- Severe pain.
- Underlying necrosis or abscess.
- Removal of infected tissue including bone involvement (i.e. osteomyelitis).
- Debulking of subcutaneous calcinosis [3].

Surgical modalities include the following:

- Digital (periarterial) sympathectomy: may benefit early digital ischemia.
- Sympathetic blocks: In patients with significant Raynaud's or risk of threatened ischemic digit.

- Stellate ganglion blocks.
- Lumbar sympathetic blocks with guanethidine.
- Local or regional sympathectomy [5].

13.5 Conclusion

Non-pharmacological measures remain the first-line therapy in both primary and secondary RP. Calcium channel blockers, specifically long-acting dihydropyridines (nifedipine or amlodipine) are the first-line drugs. Second-line agents include phosphodiesterase-5 inhibitors, prostacycline analogs, endothelin-1 receptor antagonist, topical nitrates, anti-platelet drugs, and anticoagulant drugs. Medications are generally started at the lowest effective dose and gradually titrated upward keeping in mind the benefits vs dose limiting side effects. Surgical interventions such as sympathectomy or regional blocks are generally reserved for patients with severe and complicated cases or with progression to persistent digital ischemia.

References

1. Levien TL. Advances in the treatment of Raynaud's phenomenon. Vasc Health Risk Manag. 2010;6:167–77.
2. Temprano KK. A review of Raynaud's disease. Mo Med. 2016;113(2):123–6.
3. Haque A, Hughes M. Raynaud's phenomenon. Clin Med (Lond). 2020;20(6):580–7. https://doi.org/10.7861/clinmed.2020-0754.
4. Musa R, Qurie A. Raynaud disease. In: StatPearls. StatPearls Publishing; 2022. http://www.ncbi.nlm.nih.gov/books/NBK499833/. Accessed 21 Feb 2023.
5. Pauling JD, Hughes M, Pope JE. Raynaud's phenomenon—an update on diagnosis, classification and management. Clin Rheumatol. 2019;38(12):3317–30. https://doi.org/10.1007/s10067-019-04745-5.
6. Schiopu E, Hsu VM, Impens AJ, et al. Randomized placebo-controlled crossover trial of tadalafil in Raynaud's phenomenon secondary to systemic sclerosis. J Rheumatol. 2009;36(10):2264–8. https://doi.org/10.3899/jrheum.090270.
7. Linnemann B, Erbe M. Raynaud's phenomenon and digital ischaemia—pharmacologic approach and alternative treatment options. Vasa. 2016;45(3):201–12. https://doi.org/10.1024/0301-1526/a000526.
8. Coleiro B, Marshall SE, Denton CP, Howell K, Blann A, Welsh KI, Black CM. Treatment of Raynaud's phenomenon with the selective serotonin reuptake inhibitor fluoxetine. Rheumatology (Oxford). 2001 Sep;40(9):1038–43. https://doi.org/10.1093/rheumatology/40.9.1038. PMID: 11561116.
9. Wood HM, Ernst ME. Renin—angiotensin system mediators and Raynaud's phenomenon. Ann Pharmacother. 2006;40(11):1998–2002. https://doi.org/10.1345/aph.1H201.
10. Rosato E, Borghese F, Pisarri S, Salsano F. The treatment with N-acetylcysteine of Raynaud's phenomenon and ischemic ulcers therapy in sclerodermic patients: a prospective observational study of 50 patients. Clin Rheumatol. 2009;28(12):1379–84. https://doi.org/10.1007/s10067-009-1251-7.
11. Neirotti M, Longo F, Molaschi M, Macchione C, Pernigotti L. Functional vascular disorders: treatment with pentoxifylline. Angiology. 1987;38(8):575–80. https://doi.org/10.1177/000331978703800801.

Management of Discoid Lupus Erythematosus (DLE)

14

Sudip Kumar Ghosh, Sharmistha Panja, and Partha Mukherjee

Abstract

Accurate diagnosis and effective management of discoid lupus erythematosus are critical to prevent irreversible disfigurement and potential progression to systemic lupus erythematosus (SLE). The management begins with a thorough clinical assessment and system screening. General management emphasizes strict photoprotection and supportive care. Topical therapies—including potent corticosteroids, calcineurin inhibitors, and retinoids—serve as the first-line treatment for localized disease. For extensive or refractory cases, systemic therapies such as antimalarials, corticosteroids, immunosuppressants, and biologics are employed. Surgical modalities, including excision and laser therapy, may be considered for residual scarring. Regular monitoring of disease activity and treatment-related adverse effects is essential to achieving optimal outcomes.

Keywords

Potent corticosteroids · Tacrolimus · Hydroxychloroquine

This chapter will outline management of discoid lupus erythematosus (DLE) with focus on investigations that would help to confirm the diagnosis, assess prognosis, and guide pharmacotherapy.

S. K. Ghosh (✉) · S. Panja
Department of Dermatology, Venereology, & Leprosy, R.G. Kar Medical College, Kolkata, India

P. Mukherjee
Department of Dermatology, Venereology, & Leprosy, College of Medicine & JNM Hospital, Kalyani, West Bengal, India

P. Agarwal et al. (eds.), *Dermatologist's Handbook of Autoimmune Connective Tissue Diseases*, https://doi.org/10.1007/978-981-95-0524-1_14

14.1 Investigations

Thorough clinical history and physical examination guide the physician for testing of appropriate system. Figure 14.1 shows the workflow to reach a diagnosis in a DLE patient and screening of commonly involved systems. A detailed review of investigations in a DLE patient can be found in Chap. 4.

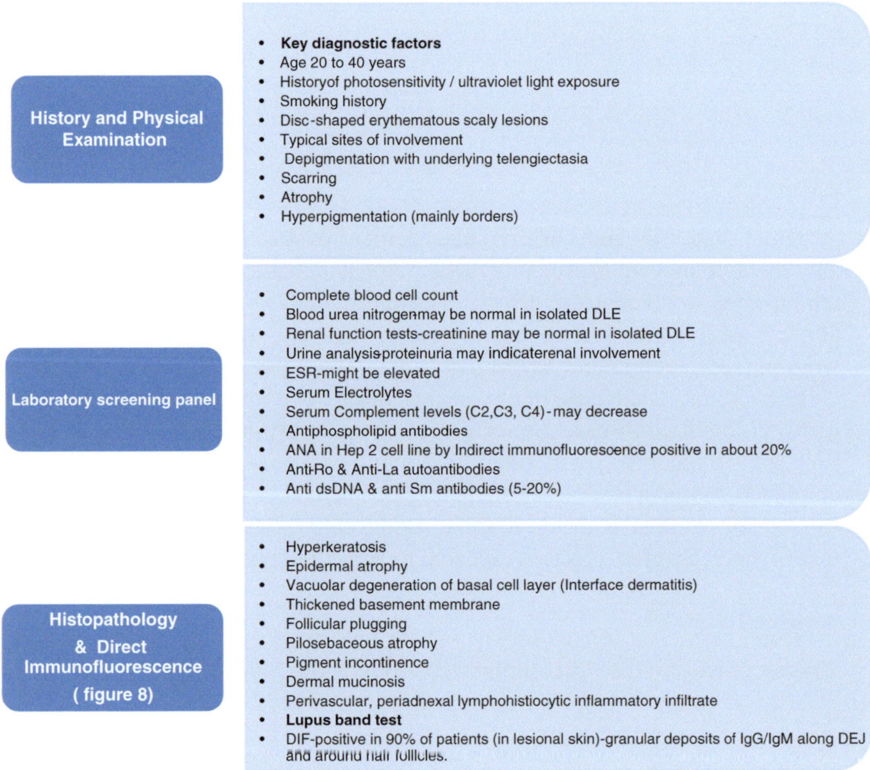

Fig. 14.1 Stepwise diagnostic approach of DLE

14.2 Treatment [1–5]

- To control disease activity (thereby preventing scarring and the development of further lesions).
- Patients should be informed that serious systemic illness may develop, albeit infrequently.
- Routine clinical assessments, including a comprehensive review of symptoms along with basic laboratory tests such as complete blood count, renal function analysis, and urinalysis, are typically adequate for monitoring the transition from localized skin disease to systemic manifestations.

14.2.1 General Measures

- Photo protection: Therapy begins with the use of sun-protective measures, including broad-spectrum sunscreens, photo protective clothing, wide-brimmed hats, and behavior alteration.
- Avoidance of isomorphic trigger factors.
- Vitamin D supplementation.
- Cessation of smoking (active and passive).
- It is better to avoid hormonal contraception containing estrogen and estrogen replacement therapy.
- Cosmetic measures, such as cover-up makeup or wigs, may be suggested for appropriately selected patients.

14.2.2 Standard Topical Medical Therapy

14.2.2.1 Topical Corticosteroids

Super high-potency (super potent ultra-high) or high-potency corticosteroids like clobetasol propionate (0.05%), fluocinonide cream (0.05%), halobetasol propionate (0.05%) cream, and betamethasone dipropionate ointment (0.05%) are recommended for twice-daily application. They are often the primary approach for managing discoid lupus erythematosus (DLE), impacting both B and T cells, reducing immunoglobulins, and suppressing TNF-alpha production. However, due to well-documented side effects such as skin atrophy, telangiectasia, and steroid-induced rosacea-like dermatitis, treatment with topical corticosteroids should be intermittent and limited to a few weeks' duration. For patients with extensive disease or a risk of scarring, concurrent therapy with antimalarials is advised.

14.2.2.2 Topical Calcineurin Inhibitors

Topical calcineurin inhibitors, including pimecrolimus (1%) cream and tacrolimus (0.03% or 0.1%) ointment applied twice daily, have also been utilized in DLE patients. They work by decreasing or blocking cytokine production from activated T lymphocytes. In active, edematous CLE lesions, particularly those on the face,

0.1% tacrolimus ointment may be considered as an alternative first-line or second-line topical treatment option.

14.2.2.3 Topical Retinoids

Topical retinoids have shown promise, particularly in hypertrophic discoid lupus erythematosus (DLE), by promoting collagen synthesis and epidermal turnover and by inhibiting melanogenesis and inflammation. Examples include 0.05% tazarotene gel, 0.025% tretinoin gel, 0.05% tretinoin cream, or tocoretinate ointment, a synthetic esterified compound combining tocopherol and retinoic acid, which can be employed as topical therapies. Their efficacy has been demonstrated in treating resistant cases of cutaneous lupus erythematosus (CLE), particularly in hypertrophic DLE lesions.

14.3 Intralesional Injections

Intralesional corticosteroid-like triamcinolone acetonide (3–5 mg/mL) has also been used.

14.4 Systemic Therapy

14.4.1 Antimalarials

Antimalarials, including hydroxychloroquine sulfate (HCQ), with chloroquine (CQ) and quinacrine as potential alternatives, are recommended as the primary and extended systemic treatment for patients with discoid lupus erythematosus (DLE) presenting with severe or extensive skin lesions, especially in those at risk of scarring and systemic disease progression.

A starting dose of 200 mg/day of hydroxychloroquine (HCQ) is recommended, with a potential increase to 200 mg twice daily after 1–2 weeks if the patient tolerates the medication well. The dosage of HCQ should not exceed 5 mg/kg of body weight per day, and tapering to 200 mg/day is typically adequate for maintenance therapy. Chloroquine may be substituted for HCQ for a subset of patients who respond preferentially to this drug. Its dose should be $\leq$2.3 mg/kg body weight per day. It's important to note that CQ and HCQ should never be concurrently prescribed due to the risk of additive side effects. In cases where monotherapy with HCQ proves ineffective, quinacrine can be added at a daily dose of 100 mg.

Ophthalmological assessment is recommended for all cutaneous lupus erythematosus (CLE) patients treated with HCQ or CQ at the outset, with subsequent annual evaluations after 5 years of treatment initiation or sooner if risk factors are present.

14.4.2 Systemic Corticosteroids

In cases of severe or extensive active lesions, systemic corticosteroids are advised as the initial treatment alongside antimalarials. The typical oral dosage of systemic corticosteroids is 0.5–1 mg of prednisolone per kilogram of body weight daily for approximately 2–4 weeks, followed by a gradual reduction to a minimum dosage (≤7.5 mg/day) with the objective of discontinuation as soon as feasible due to their recognized adverse effects.

14.4.3 Immune Suppressants and Miscellaneous Drugs

For recalcitrant disease, immunosuppressants and immunomodulators, including methotrexate, mycophenolate mofetil, azathioprine, and thalidomide, among others, may be considered.

- *Methotrexate:* Typical dose for DLE ranges from 10 to 25 mg per week, with an initial dose of 10 mg per week for adult. If the laboratory results are normal, the dose of methotrexate may be increased by 5 mg every 2 weeks up to a maximum dose of 25 mg per week.
- *Oral retinoids* such as acitretin and isotretinoin are used for DLE at a dose of 0.2–1 mg/kg/day.
- *Mycophenolate mofetil* is given in doses of 1–3 g per day in two divided doses. Treatment is usually started at 500 mg twice daily and subsequently can be increased up to 1.5 g twice daily.
- *Dapsone* has variable efficacy in the treatment of DLE and SCLE. Its therapeutic dose ranges from 25 to 200 mg daily in adults. Treatment is initiated with low doses (50 mg per day), and the dose is gradually increased while closely monitoring hematologic parameters with a maximum dose not exceeding 1.5 mg/kg.
- *Azathioprine:* DLE patients with normal thiopurine methyltransferase (TPMT) activity may be treated with a dose of 1–2.5 mg/kg/day particularly in refractory cases and with systemic involvement.
- *Thalidomide* should be initiated at doses of 50–100 mg/day and tapered to the lowest effective dose. Doses of 25–50 mg/day or less can be given as maintenance therapy. Due to potential teratogenic effect, this drug must be avoided in women of child-bearing potential.
- *Lenalidomide* is a thalidomide derivative and is used at a dose of 5–10 mg per day in adults.
- *Intravenous immune globulin (IVIG)* is often administered at a dose of 2 g/kg every 4–8 weeks depending upon response.

14.5 Surgical Modalities [6, 7]

- Excision of burned out, scarred lesions may be done.

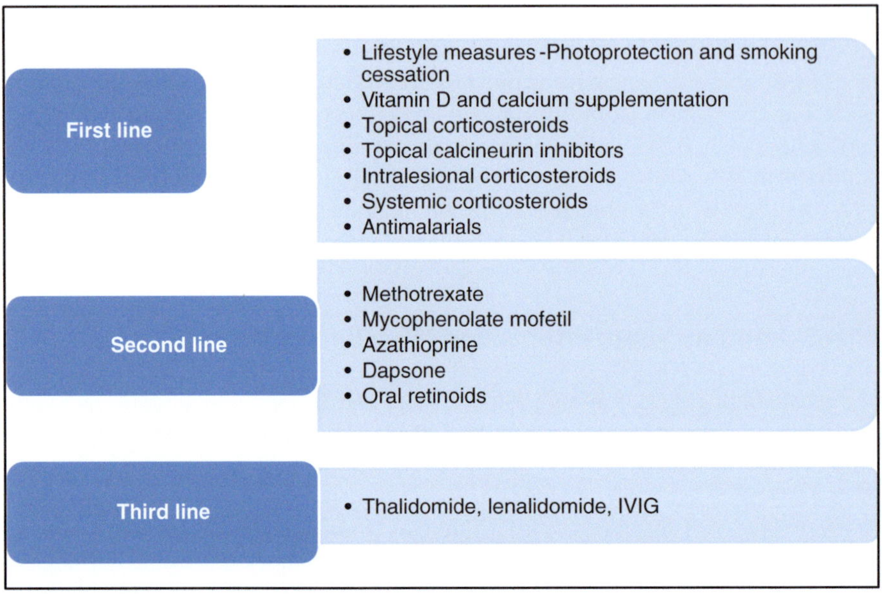

Fig. 14.2 Step-wise medical management of DLE

- Laser therapy may be useful for lesions with prominent telangiectasias. However, reactivation of inactive lesions may occur with these therapeutic modalities.

Periodic assessment of DLE lesions and monitoring of therapy-related side effects is essential to avoid complications and promote clinical resolution. The management of DLE is summarized in Fig. 14.2.

14.6 Conclusion

Management strategies of discoid lupus erythematosus must be individualized, combining general measures, topical therapies, and systemic agents based on disease severity and response. Photoprotection, lifestyle modification, and patient education remain cornerstone interventions. While topical corticosteroids and antimalarials form the foundation of therapy, immunosuppressants and biologics may be necessary for refractory or extensive disease. Surgical options can offer cosmetic improvement in selected cases. Long-term follow-up and vigilance for therapy-related adverse effects are essential for optimizing outcomes and enhancing quality of life in patients with DLE.

References

1. O'Kane D, McCourt C, Meggitt S, et al. British Association of Dermatologists guidelines for the management of people with cutaneous lupus erythematosus 2021. Br J Dermatol. 2021;185(6):1112–23.
2. Kuhn A, Aberer E, Bata-Csörgő Z, et al. S2k guideline for treatment of cutaneous lupus erythematosus – guided by the European Dermatology Forum (EDF) in cooperation with the European Academy of Dermatology and Venereology (EADV). J Eur Acad Dermatol Venereol. 2017;31(3):389–404.
3. Wahie S, Daly AK, Cordell HJ, et al. Clinical and pharmacogenetic influences on response to hydroxychloroquine in discoid lupus erythematosus: a retrospective cohort study. J Invest Dermatol. 2011;131(10):1981–6.
4. Hannon CW, McCourt C, Lima HC, Chen S, Bennett C. Interventions for cutaneous disease in systemic lupus erythematosus. Cochrane Database Syst Rev. 2021;3(3):CD007478.
5. Nahmias Z, Nambudiri VE, Vleugels RA. Thalidomide and lenalidomide for the treatment of refractory dermatologic conditions. J Am Acad Dermatol. 2016;75(1):210–2.
6. Joseph AK, Abbas LF, Chong BF. Treatments for disease damage in cutaneous lupus erythematosus: a narrative review. Dermatol Ther. 2021;34(5):e15034.
7. Flood K, Blankenship DW, Valentin M, DeWitt C. Treatment of discoid lupus erythematosus with pulsed dye laser. J Am Acad Dermatol. 2017;76(6):AB265.

Management of Systemic Lupus Erythematosus

15

Kabir Sardana, Siddharth Gogate, and Ashish Jagati

Abstract

Systemic lupus erythematosus (SLE) is a chronic autoimmune condition characterized by myriad clinical manifestations and an unpredictable disease course, which demands multidisciplinary treatment approach. Management strategies include lifestyle modifications, topical and systemic therapies, and biologics. General measures such as photoprotection, exercise, smoking cessation, and vaccinations are important in disease control and flare prevention. Treatment strategies now follow a treat-to-target approach, aiming for disease remission while minimizing treatment-related toxicity. This chapter summarizes current therapeutic options in SLE, integrating conventional and emerging therapies.

Keywords

Biological drugs · Immunomodulatory imide drugs (IMiDs) · Systemic lupus erythematosus

K. Sardana (✉) · S. Gogate
PGIMER, Dr. Ram Manohar Lohia Hospital, New Delhi, India

A. Jagati
Department of Skin & VD, Smt SCL General Hospital, Smt NHL Municipal Medical College, Ahmedabad, Gujarat, India

P. Agarwal et al. (eds.), *Dermatologist's Handbook of Autoimmune Connective Tissue Diseases*, https://doi.org/10.1007/978-981-95-0524-1_15

15.1 Introduction

SLE follows an unpredictable course, and its management is essentially multidisciplinary. As with other AICTDs, the management comprises of general measures and organ-specific measures which overlap to a large extent. Treatment of lupus should be based on regular assessments of (1) disease activity, (2) damage, (3) quality of life (and other patient reported outcomes), (4) comorbidities, and (5) drug toxicity.

A "treat to target" principle was introduced in 2014 regarding the various treatment strategies.

15.2 Investigations [1, 2, 3]

In a suspected case of systemic lupus erythematous, laboratory investigations can aid in the diagnosis. Initial investigations should serve the purpose of screening, which are then followed by investigations to confirm the diagnosis and to look for organ damage and complications. These will help in management and give an insight about the prognosis as well. Relevant investigations are summarized in Table 15.1.

Table 15.1 Investigations for initial screening, for monitoring, organ-specific diagnostic test

Initial (in suspected case)	Monitoring test in follow-up	Organ-specific diagnostic test as and when required
Complete blood count: Anemia, leukopenia, lymphopenia, thrombocytopenia, prolonged partial activated thromboplastin (aPTT) **ESR and CRP**: Elevated in both SLE flare and infection **ESR: CRP** provides diagnostic value **Liver function test**: Can be elevated in acute SLE **Urine analysis**: Low serum albumin, persistent proteinuria, red and white cell cast **Antinuclear antibodies (ANA)** (using HEp2 cell to see pattern) **[discussed in Chap. 3]** **In a positive screening test and ANA** Autoantibodies and extractable nuclear antigen antibodies (ENAs) 24-h urine protein level, spot protein/spot creatinine ratio Serum creatinine Liver function test: can be elevated in acute SLE Complement level: low C3 and C4 in active SLE Coombs test Antiphospholipid antibodies, lupus anticoagulant Creatine kinase level: Increase in myositis and overlap syndromes Lactate dehydrogenase (LDH) Ferritin: Often elevated in macrophage activation syndrome (MAS) Thyroid function test: Autoimmune thyroid abnormality can be seen Renal biopsy (presence of persistent proteinuria ≥0.5 g/24 h or UPCR ≥500 mg/g in morning first void urine)	**For SLE:** Every 3–6 months according to disease progression **For lupus nephritis** Every 2–4 weeks for the first 2–4 months after diagnosis or flare after that according to the response to therapy. Monitoring for renal and extra-renal disease activity should be life-long, at least every 3–6 months Medical history and physical examination (including bodyweight and blood pressure) Disease activity evaluation with standardized score Organ damage evaluation according to standardized score once yearly Yearly screening for comorbidity Ocular examination in patient on antimalarial – baseline then every 6 months Laboratory investigations ESR CRP Blood count with differential count Creatinine Liver enzyme Protein/creatinine ratio 24-h urine protein Urine microscopy Complement C3, C4 Anti-ds DNA Repeat renal biopsy: Useful in refractory, worsening disease, or relapse	**Mucocutaneous**: Biopsy for histopathology, immunofluorescence **Musculoskeletal**: Creatinine kinase, electromyography, magnetic resonance imaging (MRI), muscle biopsy, X-ray, arthrosonography **Renal**: Ultrasonography, renal biopsy **Cardio-pulmonary**: Chest X-ray, thoracic high-resolution computed tomography (HRCT), pulmonary function test including diffusion capacity, cardiac MRI, transesophageal echocardiography **Occular:** Funduscopy, special investigation in patients on antimalarials **Nervous system**: Electroencephalography, MRI, computed tomography, CSF analysis, carotid artery Doppler, neuropsychiatric examination, nerve conduction velocity **Gastrointestinal system**: Endoscopy, abdominal ultrasonography if indicated

15.3 General Measures [4–8]

1. **Photoprotection**
   - One of the most critical aspects of management in SLE. Given the ubiquitous exposure to UVR, repeated counselling of patients is needed to ensure compliance.
   - Given that the threshold of UV exposure required to trigger LE is far less than sunburn, it is paramount to apply sunscreen adequately.
   - A broad spectrum ≥50 SPF sunscreen applied 20 min before sun exposure is essential as flares induced by UV exposure can also affect internal organs.
   - Physical sunscreens are preferred as they have a broad-spectrum action covering both the UVB and UVA portions of the electromagnetic spectra, both of which aggravate SLE.
   - Use of broad brimmed hats or tightly woven cloth covering the face augments the sun protection. Avoidance of outdoor activities during peak sun hours (10 am–2 pm) is advisable.
2. A **dietary modification** in the form of high-protein diet is advisable to patients who have documented proteinuria.
3. **Regular exercise** improves exercise capacity, fatigue, and depressive symptoms and secondary fibromyalgia.
4. **Vascular risk factor management**: Cardiovascular risk factors like smoking, diabetes, hypertension, and hyperlipidemias must be kept in check as SLE patients are at increased risk of cardiovascular disease (CVD). Glucocorticoids increase the risk, while antimalarial have a more favorable glucose and lipid profile and display antithrombotic activity. Primary prevention with statins and aspirin should be taken into account.
5. **Vitamin D**

   Patients with SLE are at a risk for vitamin D deficiency due to sun avoidance, chronic steroid use, and renal disease. Vitamin D deficiency may slightly increase immune system hyperactivity. Hence vitamin D supplementation is warranted, with recommended doses of 1000 to 2000 q.d. or 20,000 IU once a week.
6. **Vaccinations**—The prolonged immunosuppression in SLE patients makes it advisable to give vaccines against *Streptococcus pneumoniae* (q5 years) and *Haemophilus influenzae* virus (yearly) (note that use of live vaccines may be contraindicated if they take glucocorticoids and/or immunosuppressant).
7. **Malignancy**: Women with SLE exposed to immunosuppressive drugs particularly cyclophosphamide in a cumulative dose fashion are at higher risk of cervical dysplasia likely associated with HPV. Hence, Papanicolaou (PAP) smear yearly is suggested in highly immunosuppressed individuals or according to local screening program in low-risk patients. HPV vaccination should be offered to young women with stable/inactive SLE and/or APS according to local protocols with caution in individuals with high-risk aPL profile.

15.4 Topical Management [9]

1. **Topical corticosteroids**: Moderate to high potent steroids are advised during acute flare of cutaneous lesions. They need to be tapered judiciously to prevent steroid-induced damage. Higher potency steroids can be given for a short duration even over the face in discoid lesions.
2. **Tacrolimus:** Tacrolimus 0.01% ointment serves as a good steroid sparing agent and is useful in long-term management of cutaneous lesions.

15.5 Systemic Management [10–16]

15.5.1 For Cutaneous Involvement

1. **Antimalarials**
   Antimalarials form the backbone of SLE management.
   - Hydroxychloroquine remains the ***gold standard for cutaneous lesions*** and is universally recommended for SLE patients in the absence of any contraindication. It is usually well tolerated, and if the dose does not exceed 6.5 mg/kg *ideal* body weight, then the chances of ocular toxicity are rare. The response usually takes 2–3 months; hence additional therapy with topical steroids is advisable during this period. Additional therapy with topical steroids is advisable during this period. The current American Guidelines of Ophthalmology for toxicity screening and the EULAR SLE management recommendations recommend baseline funduscopy and optical coherence tomography (OCT) and annual screening starting after 5 years, for patients on acceptable doses without risk factors.
   - Chloroquine (CQ): Chloroquine can be used at a dose of 3–4 mg/kg but is discouraged given the higher risk of retinopathy.
   - Mepacrine: Also known as quinacrine, it has an excellent ocular profile and can be added to HCQ/CQ to avoid dose-dependent toxicity. It can be utilized in a daily dose of 100–200 mg.
2. **Systemic corticosteroids**
   In cases of widespread skin lesions or acute flare of lesions, use of systemic corticosteroids helps in bringing rapid relief in the lesions. Corticosteroids are fast-acting agents and can be used as a bridge to control disease activity until the action of antimalarial sets in. The dose should be rapidly tapered to 5–7.5 mg/day or tried to be stopped completely due to the fear of avascular necrosis. They can be given as daily oral dose or monthly pulse dose. Pulse therapy is indicated in severe life-threatening disease:
   (i) Renal: Rapidly progressing glomerulonephritis, lupus nephritis grade III/IV.
   (ii) Hematological: Severe hemolytic anemia or severe immune thrombocytopenia, thrombotic thrombocytopenic purpura, macrophage activation syndrome, catastrophic antiphospholipid syndrome.

   (iii) Neuropsychiatric: Severe neuropsychiatric LE (NPSLE), e.g., transverse myelitis, demyelinating syndromes, cerebral vasculitis, acute confusional state.
   (iv) Pulmonary: Diffuse alveolar hemorrhage, acute lupus pneumonitis with rapidly progressing respiratory failure.
   (v) Cardiac: Myocarditis, severe pericarditis.
3. **Dapsone**
   Bullous lesions of SLE respond well to oral dapsone at the initial dose 50–100 mg/day (range 25–200 mg/day), but concurrent anemia may limit its use. Dapsone is the first-line drug for the management of bullous SLE, and rapid improvement is expected within hours. This can be used as an adjunct in confirming diagnosis. Other refractory cutaneous lesions of SLE rarely respond to dapsone.
4. **Immunomodulatory Imide Drugs (IMiDs)**
   These are also reserved for refractory cutaneous lesions. The newer congener lenalidomide is associated with better response and lesser adverse effects. Thalidomide has shown excellent results in the management of CLE. Factors precluding the use of thalidomide in routine practice are its teratogenic potential, as a significant number of SLE patients are women in the childbearing age group. Thalidomide may be used as an "induction" agent for severe/refractory SLE where there is a possibility of scarring, as the major adverse effect with long-term therapy is polyneuropathy.
5. **Calcineurin Inhibitors**
   Cyclosporine and systemic tacrolimus are good options for patients having cutaneous lesions and lupus nephritis.
6. **Immunosuppressants**
   Azathioprine, mycophenolate mofetil, or methotrexate has been shown to be less effective in refractory cutaneous lesions.
7. **Small Molecules**
   - **JAK inhibitors:** Tofacitinib has shown good response in the management of cutaneous LE as well causes improvement in the articular symptoms.

The use of various common drugs in systemic involvement is summarized in Table 15.2.

Biological Drugs in SLE [17]

With the advent of biological drugs, the management of SLE is changing fast. They aim at achieving disease remission and establishing self-tolerance. Though HCQs remain the first-line standard treatment for SLE, biologics are rapidly becoming drug of choice in case of multiple system involvement (Table 15.3).

There are multiple newer biologic agents which are in different phases of trial for SLE management and are summarized in Table 15.4.

The current updated EULAR recommendations 2023 for treatment are summarized below in Tables 15.6 and 15.7. General advice about sun protection, exercise, smoking cessation, balanced diet, maintain normal body weight, blood pressure, lipids, glucose, and cortisol should be given to all patients. In case of presence of

Table 15.2 Common drugs used for systemic involvement in systemic lupus erythematosus

Drugs	Dose	Systemic involvement	Adverse effects
Hydroxychloroquine	5 mg/kg (max. 6.5 mg/kg)	Musculoskeletal features, decreases thrombosis and bone destruction, reduces disease activity, improves overall survival	Premaculopathy, dose-dependent retinopathy, gastrointestinal intolerance, heart block, cardiomyopathy, hyperpigmentation, bleaching of hairs
Systemic steroids	20–30 mg/day to be tapered rapidly to reach 5–7.5 mg/day	Disease flare (cutaneous as well as systemic)	Weight gain, Cushingoid features, metabolic disturbances
Azathioprine	2–2.5 mg/kg/d ideally guided by TPMT levels	Cutaneous, lupus nephritis, lupus flares	Bone marrow suppression
Methotrexate	15–25 mg/week in combination with folic acid	Cutaneous, musculoskeletal features	Bone marrow suppression, hepatotoxicity, pulmonary toxicity, teratogenic
Mycophenolate mofetil	1–3 g/day in divided doses or 720–2160 mg of mycophenolate sodium	**Drug of choice for lupus nephritis**, also useful in recalcitrant cutaneous lesions, arthritis, hematological involvement	Gastrointestinal intolerance, bone marrow suppression, teratogenic
Cyclophosphamide	500 mg IV every 2 weekly for 6 doses	May be used for induction therapy in flares, lupus nephritis	Hemorrhagic cystitis, bladder cancer, bone marrow suppression
Intravenous immunoglobulin	2 g/kg of IVIg divided into 5 consecutive days	Lupus nephritis, thrombocytopenia, neuropsychiatric LE, myocarditis	Infusion reactions, fluid overload, thromboembolic events

aPL/APS/APS associated nephropathy acetyl salicylic acid, vitamin K antagonist acetyl salicylic acid, VKA, and heparin should be started accordingly.

Color coding is given as per grading recommendation as below (Table 15.5) **for both** Tables 15.6 and 15.7**, and the sequence of drugs does not indicate the order of preference (e.g., MTX, AZA, and MMF are all equal options for second-line therapy in mild disease or first-line therapy in moderate disease in non-renal and MMF, low-dose cyclophosphamide alone or in combination in lupus nephritis)**.

Treatment of non-renal systemic lupus erythematosus is summarized in Table 15.6 according to EULAR recommendation.

Treatment of lupus nephritis as per EULAR recommendation is summarized in Table 15.7.

Table 15.3 Biological drugs in SLE

Drug	Target	Mode of action	Indication
Rituximab	CD20	B cell targeted	Refractory SLE, lupus nephritis, neuropsychiatric LE
Belimumab	BlyS	B cell targeted	FDA approved for moderate SLE (non-responsive to HCQs, steroids) Better response in cutaneous, musculoskeletal, and neuropsychiatric features
Anifrolumab	Interferon I receptor	Antibody to interleukin 17A	FDA approved for moderate to severe SLE (without renal or neuropsychiatric features)
Secukinumab	Interleukin 17A	Interferon I receptor antagonist	Lupus nephritis
Tocilizumab	IL6		Musculoskeletal LE
Baricitinib	Janus kinase	JAK inhibitor	Refractory cutaneous LE

Table 15.4 Newer biologic agents in management of SLE [18–21]

Mechanism of action	Drugs
Monoclonal antibody against soluble and membrane bound BlyS (B lymphocyte stimulator) protein	Tabalumab, blisibimod, ianalumab Atacicept
Monoclonal antibody against CD20	Ofatumumab, ocrelizumab, obinutuzumab
Monoclonal antibody against CD38	Daratumumab
Monoclonal antibody against CD19	Obexelimab
Bruton's tyrosine kinase inhibitor	Fenebrutinib, ibrutinib
Tyrosine kinase 2 inhibitor	Deucravacitinib [11]
Polyethylene glycol-conjugated antigen-binding (fab′) fragment which targets CD40L	Dapirolizumab pegol [12]
Monoclonal antibody targeting blood dendritic cell antigen 2 (BDCA2)	Litifilimab [13]

Table 15.5 Color coding used for drugs as per grading recommendation

Grade A: Body of evidence can be trusted to guide practice
Grade B: Body of evidence can be trusted to guide practice in most situations
Grade C: Body of evidence provides some support for recommendation, (s) but care should be taken in its application

Table 15.6 Treatment of non-renal SLE

Treatment of Non-renal Systemic lupus erythematosus		
Hydroxychloroquine (HCQ) [in all patients unless contraindicated]		
GC PO/IV (if needed, short-term use to control active disease; taper to less than or 5 mg/day as early as possible and discontinue, if possible)		
Disease severity	**First line**	**Second line**
MILD Mild arthritis Rash ≤ 9% body surface area (BSA) Platelet count-50–100 $\times 10^9$/L SLEDAI ≤ 6 BILAG C ≤ 1BILAG B manifestations	Hydroxychloroquine (HCQ)	HCQ MTX MMF AZA BEL ANI
MODERATE Moderate to severe arthritis (RA like) Rash 9%–18% BSA Platelet count 20–50× $\times 10^9$/L Serositis SLEDAI –7–12 ≥ 2 BILAG B manifestations	HCQ Methotrexate (MTX) Mycophenolate mofetil (MMF) Azathioprine (AZA) Belimumab (BEL) Anifrolumab (ANI) Calcineurin inhibitor (CNI)	HCQ MMF BEL ANI CNI
SEVERE Major organ threatening diseases • Cerebritis • Myelitis • Pneumonitis • Mesenteric vasculitis Platelet count < 20 × $\times 10^{9/L}$ thrombotic thrombocytopenia like disease OR acute hemophagocytic syndrome Rash > 18% BSA SLEDAI >12 ≥ 1 BILAG A manifestations	HCQ MMF Belimumab (BEL) Anifrolumab (ANI) Cyclophosphamide (CYC) Rituximab (RTX)	HCQ CYC RTX
TARGET **Remission:** Clinical SLEDAI=0 HCQ GC ≤5 mg/dl ***OR*** **Low disease activity:** SLEDAI ≤4 HCQ GC≤5 mg/day Immunosuppressive or biological agents at stable and tolerated dose		

aPL antiphospholipid antibodies, *APS* antiphospholipid syndrome, *BILAG* British Isles Lupus Assessment Group, *GC* glucocorticoids, *IV* intravenous, *PO* per os, *SLEDAI* SLE Disease Activity Index

Table 15.7 Treatment of lupus nephritis

Treatment of Lupus Nephritis	
Adjunct treatment for renal protection ACE inhibitor/Angiotensin receptor blockers In case of decreased estimated glomerular filtration rate (eGFR)-Consider–sodium glucose transporter 2 inhibitors	
GC PO/IV (consider pulse IV methylprednisolone followed by 0.3–0.5 mg/kg/day based on severity, quickly taper to≤ 5mg / day)	
Initial	Hydroxychloroquine (HCQ)
	Mycophenolate mofetil (MMF)
	Low dose cyclophosphamide (CYC)
	MMF/Low dose CYC + belimumab (BEL)
	MMF+ CNI (calcineurin inhibitor specially voclosporin, tacrolimus)
	High-dose CYC
	Rituximab
Subsequent	Hydroxychloroquine (HCQ)
	Mycophenolate mofetil (MMF)
	Azathioprine (AZA)/MMF
	MMF/AZA +BEL
	MMF+ CNI (calcineurin inhibitor specially voclosporin, tacrolimus)
	High dose CYC
	Rituximab
• *BEL should always be given in combination with MMF or low-dose CYC as initial therapy and with MMF or AZA as maintenance therapy.* • *Calcineurin inhibitor should be given in combination with MMF* • *High-dose cyclophosphamide is Specially recommended in the presence of poor prognostic factors such as reduced eGFR, histological presence of cellular crescents or fibrinoid necrosis, or severe interstitial inflammation* • Rituximab should be used in relapse or in refractory cases (after failure to CYC-based regimens)	
Target **(with eGFR within 10% of baseline)** 3 months ≥ 25 % reduction in urine protein (UPr) 6 months ≥ reduction in UPr or ≤ 3gm/day 12–24 months–UPr ≤ 0.5–0,7 gm/day	

GC glucocortocoids, *IV* intravenous, *PO*, per os

Table 15.8 Drugs used in single organ manifestation

Treatment of systemic lupus erythematosus presented initially with single organ involved					
	Cutaneous	**Musculoskele tal**	**Nephritis**	**Hematological (Cytopenia)**	**Neuropsychia tric SLE**
First line	**Topicals** (Broad spectrumsun screen, corticosteroid, calcineurin inhibitors)	MTX BEL	MMF CYC	IVIG (if there is no response to high dose of glucocorticosteroid or rapid increase in platelet or haematocrit is needed)	CYC
Second line	MTX AZA/CsA MMF BEL		AZA	AZA MMF CsA	AZA MMF
Refractory disease	Dapsone Thalidomide Rituximab	Rituximab	Rituximab Tacrolimus BEL Voclosporin	CYC Rituximab	Rituximab
RTX is off-label and should be used in refractory disease					
Cyclosporine, azathioprine, MMF are usually not used for arthritis. In women of childbearing age group, leflunomide should be avoided due to the need for cholestyramine washout following its discontinuation.					

Majority of lupus patients present with multi-organ manifestations, and the aim is to achieve remission or low disease activity (LDA) in all the organs as per the updated EULAR recommendations. However, less than 10% of patients initially present with a single, but severe manifestation from one organ system, and treatment in these patients varies according to the presenting clinical manifestations, as summarized below in Table 15.8 [22]. HCQ is recommended in all patients irrespective of the severity and organ involved. Similarly, depending on extent and severity, systemic glucocorticosteroid can be used at moderate doses and should be reduced to 5–7.5 mg/day within 3–6 months [22].

The main targets of SLE treatment concern remission and Lupus Low Disease Activity State (LLDAS) in non-renal and renal lupus and GC reduction.

When remission cannot be reached, the target form disease activity control shifts to attaining lowest possible disease activity (Table 15.9) [23].

Table 15.9 Definition of remission and low lupus disease activity state

	DORIS (Definition Of Remission In SLE)	LLDAS (Low Lupus. Disease Activity State)
Clinical SLEDAI	0	≤4
Physician Global (0-3)	≤ 0.5	≤1
Organ involvement	No active	No new or critical active
Hydroxychloroquine	Allowed (and recommended)	Allowed (and recommended)
Glucocorticoids	≤ 5 mg prednisone q.d.	≤ 7.5 mg prednisone q.d.
Immunomodulation	Maintenance therapy	Well tolerated maintenance therapy and approved DMARDS

15.6 Conclusion

The management of systemic lupus erythematosus requires a personalized and multidisciplinary approach aimed at controlling disease activity, preventing flares, and minimizing long-term organ damage. Outcome of treatment depends on early diagnosis, patient education, adherence to therapy, and management of the comorbidities, including cardiovascular risk and infections. With timely and appropriate intervention, many patients with SLE can achieve remission or low disease activity and maintain a good quality of life.

References

1. Rasaratnam I, Ryan PFJ. 10. Systemic lupus erythematosus. Med J Aust. 1997;166(5):266–70. https://doi.org/10.5694/j.1326-5377.1997.tb140110.x.
2. Kuhn A, Bonsmann G, Anders HJ, Herzer P, Tenbrock K, Schneider M. The diagnosis and treatment of systemic lupus erythematosus. Dtsch Arztebl Int. 2015;112(25):423–32. https://doi.org/10.3238/arztebl.2015.0423.
3. Fanouriakis A, Kostopoulou M, Cheema K, et al. 2019 update of the Joint European League Against Rheumatism and European Renal Association-European Dialysis and Transplant Association (EULAR/ERA-EDTA) recommendations for the management of lupus nephritis. Ann Rheum Dis. 2020;79(6):713–23. https://doi.org/10.1136/annrheumdis-2020-216924.
4. McDonald KA, Lytvyn Y, Mufti A, Chan AW, Rosen CF. Review on photoprotection: a clinician's guide to the ingredients, characteristics, adverse effects, and disease-specific benefits of chemical and physical sunscreen compounds. Arch Dermatol Res. 2023;315:735–49.
5. O'Dwyer T, Durcan L, Wilson F. Exercise and physical activity in systemic lupus erythematosus: a systematic review with meta-analyses. Semin Arthritis Rheum. 2017;47:204–15.

6. Parodis I, Gomez A, Frodlund M, Jönsen A, Zickert A, Sjöwall C, et al. Smoking reduces the efficacy of belimumab in mucocutaneous lupus. Expert Opin Biol Ther. 2018;18:911–20.
7. Chasset F, Francès C, Barete S, Amoura Z, Arnaud L. Influence of smoking on the efficacy of antimalarials in cutaneous lupus: a meta-analysis of the literature. J Am Acad Dermatol. 2015;72:634–9.
8. Andreoli L, et al. EULAR recommendations for women's health and the management of family planning, assisted reproduction, pregnancy and menopause in patients with systemic lupus erythematosus and/or antiphospholipid syndrome. Ann Rheum Dis. 2017;76(3):476–85. https://doi.org/10.1136/annrheumdis-2016-209770.
9. Fanouriakis A, Kostopoulou M, Andersen J, Aringer M, Arnaud L, Bae SC, Boletis J, Bruce IN, Cervera R, Doria A, Dörner T. EULAR recommendations for the management of systemic lupus erythematosus: 2023 update. Ann Rheum Dis. 2024;83(1):15–29.
10. Sardana K, Sinha S, Sachdeva S. Hydroxychloroquine in dermatology and beyond: recent update. Indian Dermatol Online J. 2020;11:453–64.
11. Dima A, Jurcut C, Chasset F, Felten R, Arnaud L. Hydroxychloroquine in systemic lupus erythematosus: overview of current knowledge. Ther Adv Musculoskelet Dis. 2022;14:1759720X211073001. https://doi.org/10.1177/1759720X211073001. PMID: 35186126; PMCID: PMC8848057.
12. Contestable JJ, Edhegard KD, Meyerle JH. Bullous systemic lupus erythematosus: a review and update to diagnosis and treatment. Am J Clin Dermatol. 2014;15:517–24. https://doi.org/10.1007/s40257-014-0098-0.
13. Yuki EFN, Silva CA, Aikawa NE, Romiti R, Heise CO, Bonfa E, et al. Thalidomide and lenalidomide for refractory systemic/cutaneous lupus erythematosus treatment: a narrative review of literature for clinical practice. J Clin Rheumatol. 2021;27:248–59.
14. Hou L, Zhou P, Zhao C, Wang X, Du Y. Tofacitinib for child-onset systemic lupus erythematosus. Front Immunol. 2024;15:1457821.
15. Kuhn A, Ruland V, Bonsmann G. Cutaneous lupus erythematosus: update of therapeutic options part II. J Am Acad Dermatol. 2011;65:e195–213.
16. Binello N, Cancelli C, Passalacqua S, De Vito F, Lombardi G, Gambaro G, Manna R. Use of intravenous immunoglobulin therapy at unconventional doses in refractory fulminant systemic lupus erythematosus. Eur J Case Rep Internal Med. 2018;5(9):000934.
17. Postal M, Costallat LT, Appenzeller S. Biological therapy in systemic lupus erythematosus. Int J Rheumatol. 2012;2012:578641.
18. Bokor LA, Martyin K, Krebs M, Galajda NÁ, Meznerics FA, Szabó B, et al. Deucravacitinib shows superior efficacy and safety in cutaneous lupus erythematosus compared to various biologics and small molecules—a systematic review and meta-analysis. Autoimmun Rev. 2025;24:103723.
19. Furie RA, Bruce IN, Dörner T, Leon MG, Leszczyński P, Urowitz M, et al. Phase 2, randomized, placebo-controlled trial of dapirolizumab pegol in patients with moderate-to-severe active systemic lupus erythematosus. Rheumatology (Oxford). 2021;60:5397–407.
20. Cho SK, Vazquez T, Werth VP. Litifilimab (BIIB059), a promising investigational drug for cutaneous lupus erythematosus. Expert Opin Investig Drugs. 2023;32:345–53.
21. Burns PB, Rohrich RJ, Chung KC. The levels of evidence and their role in evidence-based medicine. Plast Reconstr Surg. 2011;128(1):305–10. https://doi.org/10.1097/PRS.0b013e318219c171. PMID: 21701348; PMCID: PMC3124652.
22. Nikolopoulos D, et al. Tailored treatment strategies and future directions in systemic lupus erythematosus. Rheumatol Int. 2022;42(8):1307–19. https://doi.org/10.1007/s00296-022-05133-0.
23. Pitsigavdaki S, Nikoloudaki M, Garantziotis P, Silvagni E, Repa A, Marangoni A, Flouri I, Avgoustidis N, Parperis K, Fanouriakis A, Govoni M. Pragmatic targets for moderate/severe SLE and their implications for clinical care and trial design: sustained DORIS or LLDAS for at least 6 months is sufficient while their attainment for at least 24 months ensures high specificity for damage-free progression. Ann Rheum Dis. 2024;83(4):464–74.

Management of Systemic Sclerosis

16

Pooja Agarwal

Abstract

Systemic sclerosis (SSc) is a complex autoimmune connective tissue disease and demands a comprehensive, multidisciplinary management approach. Early detection of internal organ involvement is crucial, and a wide array of investigations—from serological test to imaging modalities—guide towards diagnosis and prognosis. Management strategies are tailored according to the extent and severity of cutaneous and systemic involvement. This chapter outlines a structured yet adaptable approach to managing SSc, integrating conventional and novel treatments to improve patient outcomes.

Keywords

Digital ulceration, Emerging therapy · Hematopoietic stem cell transplantation (HSCT) · Cutaneous Sclerosis

16.1 Introduction

As with other AICTDs, a holistic approach is needed to manage a patient of systemic sclerosis. Management does not limit itself only to specific therapy for the disease, but also includes early detection of internal organ involvement and identification of patients who are at risk for worsening of systemic disease. Importance and implications of investigations have already been outlined in earlier chapter, so they have been written only in brief in this chapter.

P. Agarwal (✉)
Department of Skin & VD, SVPIMSR, Smt NHL Municipal Medical College, Ahmedabad, Gujarat, India

P. Agarwal et al. (eds.), *Dermatologist's Handbook of Autoimmune Connective Tissue Diseases*, https://doi.org/10.1007/978-981-95-0524-1_16

16.2 Investigations [1–5]

Though systemic sclerosis is more of a clinical diagnosis, investigations are needed to assess the systemic involvement and guidance for instituting therapy. They are summarized in Table 16.1 and discussed in detail in Chaps. 3 and 4.

Pre-treatment assessment and follow-up monitoring of systemic sclerosis patient are summarized in flowchart below in Fig. 16.1 [6–9].

Table 16.1 Investigations in systemic sclerosis

Investigation	Interpretation
CBC with ESR	Anaemia, raised ESR
Renal function test	Raised blood urea, serum creatinine
Liver function test	As a baseline value before starting treatment
Urine examination (including routine microscopy and 24 h urinary protein)	For sediments and proteinuria
Skin biopsy for histopathology	Atrophic epidermis with densely packed collagen in the dermis which is oriented horizontally
ANA and ENA	Speckled pattern seen on IIF, anti-centromere, anti-topoisomerase, anti-PMSCL, anti-U3RNP
Pulmonary function test (PFT)	Shows Restrictive pattern with decrease of forced vital capacity (FVC) or total lung capacity (TLC) and DLCO even when the radiology is normal. (DLCO <10–40% 5-year survival versus >40–75% 5-year survival)
Chest X-ray and high-resolution computerized tomography (HRCT)	*Earliest finding*: diffuse reticular branching pattern in the lower zones extending from the cardiac borders towards the periphery **HRCT is gold standard**
ECG and ECHO	Arrhythmias and evidence of pulmonary arterial hypertension (PAH)
Right heart catheterization (RHC) (if required)	**Gold standard** for diagnosis of PAH (allows differentiation between pre- and post-capillary pulmonary hypertension by measuring pulmonary capillary wedge pressure which should not exceed 15 mm Hg under normal conditions)
Barium studies	Dilated atonic lower oesophagus/dilated stomach/dilated atonic colon with multiple colonic diverticula on inferior surface, predominantly in transverse and descending colon
Upper gastrointestinal endoscopy (if required)	Reflux oesophagitis and gastric antral vascular ectasia (GAVE) (appearance of a watermelon stomach)
Ultrasonography of abdomen	Dilated stomach and bowel loops
Radiological evaluation of hands and joints (if required)	Acro-osteolysis, flexion contractures of fingers and soft tissue calcinosis, osteoarthritis-like changes. MRI is sensitive in detecting synovitis and tenosynovitis

DETERMINE DISEASE SUBSET [with the help of criteria (ACR/EULAR)

Diffuse cutaneous systemic sclerosis

Limited cutaneous systemic sclerosis

Systemic sclerosis sine scleroderma

Determine the duration of the disease progression (first symptom other than Raynaud's -<3 years or >3 years)

⬇

Pre-treatment Assessment

History
Physical examination (Including modified Rodnan skin Score)
Initial Baseline investigation including Blood pressure, ECG, Echocardiogram
ANA and ENA
Pulmonary function test (with DLCO), Initial HRCT
Urine analysis
Routine monitoring of creatinine level, creatinine clearance
In case of gastrointestinal symptom- imaging tests.

⬇

Follow up monitoring

- If polymerase III antibodies present or recent diffuse cutaneous form of SSc – routine self-monitoring of blood pressure at least 3 times per week for the first 3-5 years, routine monitoring of blood creatinine levels, creatinine clearance.
- PFT with DLCO every 6 month for first 3-5 year especially Diffuse interstitial lung disease otherwise yearly.
- ECG and echocardiogram every year
- Reduced PFT result or new respiratory symptom – repeat thoracic CT
- Right heart catheterisation - in case of suspected pulmonary hypertension
- In case of suspected cardiac damage - Cardiac MRI
- Barrett's oesophagus if detected – Endoscopic screening every 3 monthly in high grade dysplasia, yearly in low grade dysplasia and 3 yearly in case of lack of dysplasia

Fig. 16.1 Pre-treatment assessments and follow-up monitoring in systemic sclerosis

16.3 Treatment [7, 10–14]

The complex nature of systemic sclerosis with variable multisystem involvement prevents from forming standardized guidelines for the treatment. The therapy is mostly directed by the extent and severity of cutaneous and systemic involvement. Other factors which affect decision-making include the current activity and duration of the disease, gender (male patients have higher chances of progression of interstitial lung disease) and autoantibody profile (anti-centromere antibodies are associated with greater chances of ILD). In this chapter we will be discussing the management of cutaneous sclerosis as detailed management of gastrointestinal, renal and pulmonary involvement is done better by the specialist consultants, but an overview is given at the end of the chapter.

16.3.1 General Measures

A patient with systemic sclerosis benefits as much from some general measures as from specific therapy. These measures aim at decreasing the morbidity due to Raynaud's phenomenon, gastrointestinal and cutaneous complaints.

- Wearing warm gloves and shoes in winters.
- Avoidance of stress, smoking, cold and trauma.
- Regular use of emollients to decrease the discomfort caused by friction and stretching of skin and avoidance of irritating or drying substances.
- Physiotherapy to help maintain functional ability, muscle strength, joint movement while preventing joint contractures.
- Frequent small meals (instead of large meals).
- Avoidance of spicy, oily food and alcohol (heartburn), fatty foods and chocolate (reduce lower oesophageal sphincter pressure).
- Avoid sympathomimetic drugs and caffeine.
- Last meal 2 h prior to going to sleep.
- Slight elevation of head end of bed.

16.3.2 Specific Therapies

The pharmacological management of systemic sclerosis is challenging as no drug has been shown to be of unequivocal benefit. Therapy can be directed as:

1. *Disease-modifying therapy*, directed at controlling the underlying disease process (immunomodulatory and antifibrotic agents).
2. *Organ-targeted therapy*, directed towards complications in involved organs.

It's important to tailor the therapeutic approach based on the individual patient's disease presentation and the extent of organ involvement.

Management of Raynaud's phenomenon has been in Chap. 13, and this section focuses on cutaneous sclerosis. The natural history of cutaneous involvement is a slow gradual improvement over years, but early treatment with immunosuppressant drugs leads to a greater reduction in skin tightening with improved psychological and body image concerns. Systemic therapies are indicated in all cases with diffuse cutaneous systemic sclerosis. mRSS forms an important tool to judge the effect of the therapy on cutaneous sclerosis and should ideally be done by the same examiner at every visit to avoid inter-observer variability.

16.3.2.1 Methotrexate

EULAR guidelines for the treatment of systemic sclerosis were updated in 2016 and have suggested methotrexate as the first line of management in cutaneous sclerosis. It appears to work best in early cases of systemic sclerosis with significant improvement in mRSS over a 12-month period. Doses studied are lower than that used in rheumatoid arthritis (10–15 mg/week intramuscular or subcutaneous). Methotrexate has not been found to have any beneficial effect on systemic involvement. Safety concerns are there for adverse effect profile ranging from pancytopenia and liver toxicity to potential for causing pulmonary fibrosis.

16.3.2.2 Mycophenolate Mofetil

More recent systematic reviews have considered mycophenolate mofetil (MMF) as a preferred choice for treatment of cutaneous sclerosis in refractory disease or in the case of intolerance in view of its safety profile. The therapy is started at 500 mg twice a day and can be safely increased till 1.5 g twice a day if the need arises. Significant reduction in mRSS and pulmonary functions have been reported over 2 years of therapy, and the effect seems to sustain beyond that also.

16.3.2.3 Cyclophosphamide

In cases which do not show much improvement with MMF, cyclophosphamide is the preferred drug. It has shown to slow down the cutaneous sclerosis and is particularly helpful in patients with progressive pulmonary disease. Both oral dosage (1–2mkg/kg/day) and monthly infusions (750 mg/m2/month initially for 6 months) have been seen to improve the mRSS as well as pulmonary function after 12 months of therapy. Maintenance dose of <1 mg/kg/day is advised for further 12 months. The caveat remains that effect of cyclophosphamide wanes after completion of maintenance therapy, and possibility of progression remains. The other limitations include unfavourable short- (leucopaenia and infections) and long-term toxicity (infertility, carcinogenesis, bone marrow toxicity). To prevent haemorrhagic cystitis, adequate hydration and frequent voiding are emphasized.

16.3.2.4 Hematopoietic Stem Cell Transplant (HSCT)

Consisting of immunoablation followed by reconstitution with autologous hematopoietic stem cell transplant is another possible therapeutic option which provides the most dramatic improvement in cutaneous sclerosis. However, its use is limited to only those cases which are refractory to immunomodulatory therapies and rapidly progressive SSc at risk of organ failure. High morbidity and mortality due to treatment-related side effects and requirement of experienced centres limit its use in management of SSc.

16.3.3 Emerging Therapies [15, 16]

Many molecules are emerging as potential candidates for halting the progression of systemic sclerosis.

16.3.3.1 Antifibrotic Agents

Pirfenidone is a synthetic agent which is FDA approved for treatment of idiopathic pulmonary fibrosis. It inhibits TGFb production and myofibroblast proliferation which suggests its potential efficacy in cutaneous sclerosis. Although it has been tried in combination with immunosuppressive medicines only, tolerability remains a major issue.

16.3.3.2 Cannabinoid Receptor Agonists

These reduce gene expressions involved in fibrotic pathways and hence may be useful in cutaneous sclerosis. Lenabasum is a selective type 2 cannabinoid receptor agonist and has been seen to be useful in reducing mRSS in early cases of dcSSc after a 16-week course with minimal adverse effects.

16.3.3.3 Biologics

Various biologic drugs are undergoing trials for producing improvement in mRSS by targeting the B cells or chemokines involved in the pathogenesis (Table 16.2).

16.3.4 Digital Ulceration [17, 18]

Finger-tip ulcers cause significant physical and psychological morbidity to the patients with SSc. Though the general measures for Raynaud's phenomenon are effective in the management of digital ulcers also, once the ulcers develop, they require targeted therapy.

- *Calcium channel blockers* (CCBs) may prevent formation of ulcers by virtue of their vasodilating properties (0.2 mg/kg every 8 h, progressively increased to 0.3 mg/kg depending on efficacy and side effects, up to a maximum of 10 mg/dose). Topical treatment is mandatory in the treatment of SSc-related digital ulcers.

Table 16.2 Biologics in systemic sclerosis

Drug	Target	Dose	Effect on mRSS
Rituximab	CD20	2 doses of 1 g 15 days apart	Favourable
Romilkimab	IL4, IL 13	2 mg subcutaneous weekly for 24 weeks	Favourable
Tocilizumab	IL 6	162 mg subcutaneous weekly for 24–28 weeks	Favourable
Abatacept	B/T cell interaction	125 mg subcutaneous weekly for 1 year	No significant change
Belimumab	Soluble form of B cell stimulating protein	10 mg/kg IV 2-weekly for the first Three doses and then 4-weekly (52 weeks)	No significant change
Nintedanib	Tyrosine kinase inhibitor	150 mg twice a day (52 weeks)	No change

- *Prostacyclins:* For established ulcers prostacyclins are the drug of choice. Intravenous iloprost is given as a 3 day/5 day or continuous infusion (0.5 and 2.0 ng/kg/min, availability is a limitation) depending on the severity of vasospasm and ulceration. Recently a synthetic prostacyclin analogue Treprostinil has been seen to be effective in healing the digital ulcers in both oral and topical formulations.
- *Phosphodiesterase 5 (PDE5) inhibitors*: Sildenafil (50 mg twice a day) and tadalafil (20 mg on alternate day) are effective in healing of existing ulcers as well as prevent new ulcers.
- *Endothelin receptor antagonists (ERA)*: Bosentan has been found effective in reducing the formation of new ulcers in which CCBs, iloprost or PDE5 inhibitors fail or are contraindicated but do not treat existing digital ulcers.

16.3.5 Calcinosis Cutis [19]

Calcinosis cutis always poses a challenge to the treating physician because of resistance as well as lack of treatment options. Low-dose warfarin and calcium channel blockers have been seen to provide some respite. Surgical removal of the calcified lesion remains the only feasible therapeutic option in patients with debilitating calcinosis hampering with quality of life to prevent recurrence or discharging fistulae. Other modalities such as bisphosphonates, minocycline, aluminium hydroxide, probenecid, ceftriaxone, colchicine, sodium thiosulfate, infliximab, IvIg, abatacept and intralesional steroid can be used. Diclofenac is a useful non-steroidal to help inflammation around calcinotic deposits. Flucloxacillin can help secondary infection that may prolong or worsen calcinosis.

16.4 Systemic Involvement and Management of Individual System [20]

A vigilant approach helps in early diagnosis of systemic involvement in systemic sclerosis patients with timely referral to specialist consultants for prompt management. A brief overview of **EULAR recommendations** for management is summarized in Fig. 16.2.

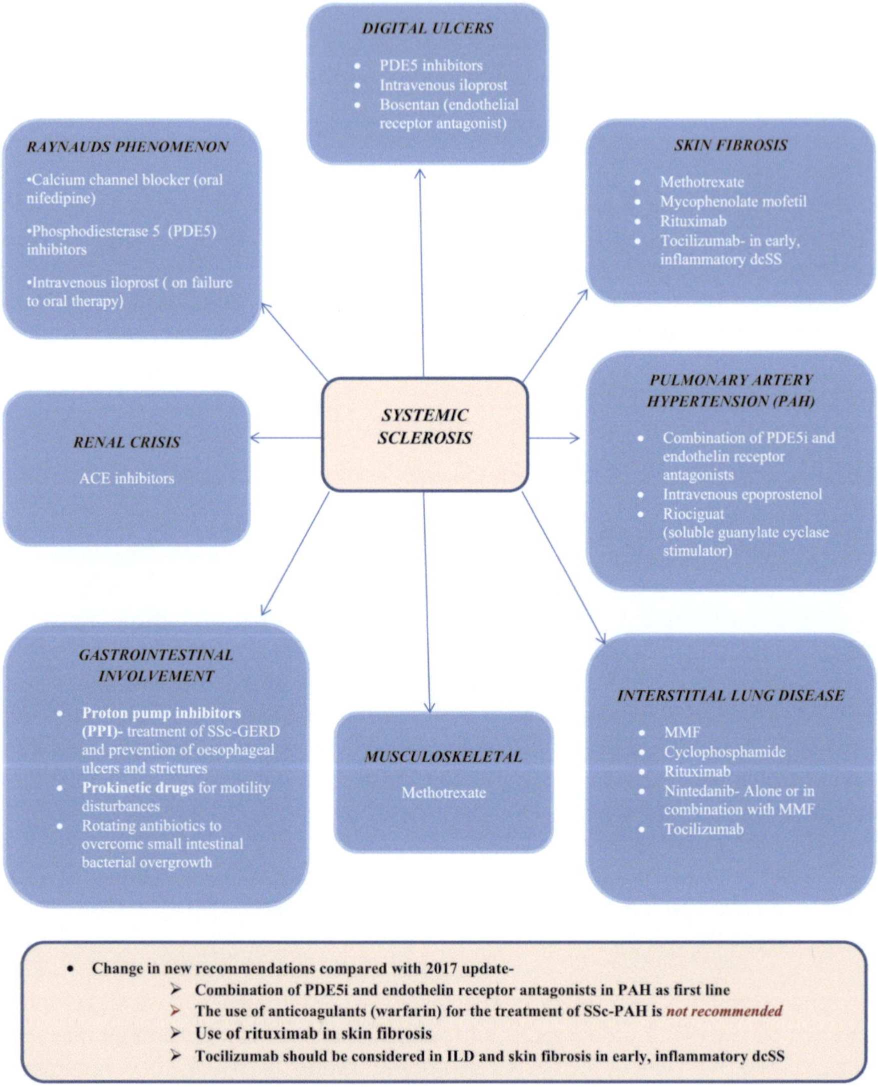

Fig. 16.2 Organ-specific management in systemic sclerosis

16.5 Conclusion

Systemic sclerosis, a complex, multisystem autoimmune disorder, needs a multidisciplinary and individualized approach for management. Early detection of organ involvement plays a crucial role in management. General measures provide symptomatic relief. The management of cutaneous sclerosis primarily relies on disease-modifying immunosuppressive therapies. Advanced treatment options like hematopoietic stem cell transplant and emerging biologics offer hope in refractory cases. Regular follow-up and monitoring for systemic complications remain crucial, with timely referral to appropriate specialists to prevent irreversible damage and improve quality of life.

References

1. Adigun R, Goyal A, Hariz A. Systemic sclerosis (scleroderma) [Updated 2024 Apr 5]. In: StatPearls [Internet]. Treasure Island: StatPearls Publishing; 2025. Available from: https://www.ncbi.nlm.nih.gov/books/NBK430875/
2. Hoffmann-Vold AM, Maher TM, Philpot EE, Ashrafzadeh A, Distler O. Assessment of recent evidence for the management of patients with systemic sclerosis-associated interstitial lung disease: a systematic review. ERJ Open Res. 2021;7(1):00235–2020. https://doi.org/10.1183/23120541.00235-2020. PMID: 33644224; PMCID: PMC7897846.
3. Chatzinikolaou SL, Quirk B, Murray C, Planche K. Radiological findings in gastrointestinal scleroderma. J Scleroderma Relat Disord. 2020;5(1):21–32. https://doi.org/10.1177/2397198319848550. Epub 2019 May 20. PMID: 35382407; PMCID: PMC8922595.
4. Showalter K, Gordon JK. Skin histology in systemic sclerosis: a relevant clinical biomarker. Curr Rheumatol Rep. 2021;23:1–8.
5. Andersen MJ, Husted A, Clemmensen TS, Olesen AB, Baumgartner J, Mellemkjær S. Pulmonary vascular dysfunction in systemic sclerosis. JHLT Open. 2024;3:100024.
6. Hachulla E, Agard C, Allanore Y, Avouac J, Bader-Meunier B, Belot A, Berezne A, Bouthors AS, Condette-Wojtasik G, Constans J, De Groote P. French recommendations for the management of systemic sclerosis. Orphanet J Rare Dis. 2021;16:1–61.
7. Bukiri H, Volkmann ER. Current advances in the treatment of systemic sclerosis. Curr Opin Pharmacol. 2022;64:102211.
8. Ariani A, Aiello M, Silva M, et al. Quantitative CT indexes are significantly associated with exercise oxygen desaturation in interstitial lung disease related to systemic sclerosis. Clin Respir J. 2017;11:983–9.
9. Denton CP, Khanna D. Systemic sclerosis. Lancet. 2017;390(10103):1685–99. https://doi.org/10.1016/S0140-6736(17)30933-9.
10. Sultan N, Pope JE, Clements PJ. The health assessment questionnaire (HAQ) is strongly predictive of good outcome in early diffuse scleroderma: results from an analysis of two randomized controlled trials in early diffuse scleroderma. Rheumatology. 2004;43(4):472–8.
11. Tashkin DP, Elashoff R, Clements PJ, Goldin J, Roth MD, Furst DE, Arriola E, Silver R, Strange C, Bolster M, Seibold JR. Cyclophosphamide versus placebo in scleroderma lung disease. N Engl J Med. 2006;354(25):2655–66.
12. Tashkin DP, Roth MD, Clements PJ, Furst DE, Khanna D, Kleerup EC, Goldin J, Arriola E, Volkmann ER, Kafaja S, Silver R. Mycophenolate mofetil versus oral cyclophosphamide in scleroderma-related interstitial lung disease (SLS II): a randomised controlled, double-blind, parallel group trial. Lancet Respir Med. 2016;4(9):708–19.
13. Rodrigues MC, Hamerschlak N, de Moraes DA, et al. Guidelines of the Brazilian society of bone marrow transplantation on hematopoietic stem cell transplantation as a treatment for the autoimmune diseases systemic sclerosis and multiple sclerosis. Rev Bras Hematol Hemoter. 2013;35:134–43.
14. Kersten BE, den Broeder N, van den Hoogen FHJ, Knaapen-Hans HAK, van den Ende CHM, Vonk MC. Treatment with cyclophosphamide IV pulse therapy is an option for effective treatment of skin fibrosis in patients with early systemic sclerosis. Rheumatology. 2020;59(7):1550–5. https://doi.org/10.1093/rheumatology/kez487.

15. Gonzalez EG, Selvi E, Balistreri E, Akhmetshina A, Palumbo K, Lorenzini S, Lazzerini PE, Montilli C, Capecchi PL, Lucattelli M, Baldi C. Synthetic cannabinoid ajulemic acid exerts potent antifibrotic effects in experimental models of systemic sclerosis. Ann Rheum Dis. 2012;71(9):1545–51.
16. Campochiaro C, Allanore Y. An update on targeted therapies in systemic sclerosis based on a systematic review from the last 3 years. Arthritis Res Ther. 2021;23(1):1–4.
17. McMahan ZH, Volkmann ER. An update on the pharmacotherapeutic options and treatment strategies for systemic sclerosis. Expert Opin Pharmacother. 2020;21(16):2041–56.
18. Le C, Bedocs PM. Calcinosis cutis. [Updated 2023 Jul 10]. In: StatPearls [Internet]. Treasure Island: StatPearls Publishing; 2025. Available from: https://www.ncbi.nlm.nih.gov/books/NBK448127/
19. Ingegnoli F, Schioppo T, Allanore Y, Caporali R, Colaci M, Distler O, Furst DE, Hunzelmann N, Iannone F, Khanna D, Matucci-Cerinic M. Practical suggestions on intravenous iloprost in Raynaud's phenomenon and digital ulcer secondary to systemic sclerosis: systematic literature review and expert consensus. Semi Arthritis rheum. 2019;48(4):686–93.
20. Del Galdo F, Lescoat A, Conaghan PG, et al. Ann Rheum Dis Epub ahead of print. https://doi.org/10.1136/ard-2024-226430.

Management of Morphea

17

Sudip Kumar Ghosh, Partha Mukherjee,
and Sharmistha Panja

Abstract

The primary aims of treatment of morphea are to halt the disease progression and prevention of new lesion development. The management is tailored according to individual person with respect to the severity, extent, and activity of the disease. While topical therapies are preferred for superficial and localized disease, rapidly progressive or deep lesions warrant use of systemic modalities. Systemic modalities encompass immunosuppression with systemic corticosteroids, methotrexate, or mycophenolate mofetil augmented with phototherapy. Surgical intervention becomes useful in the case of deformities induced by sclerotic or atrophic stage of the disease.

Keywords

Calcipotriol · Corticosteroids · Morphea

17.1 Investigations [1–3]

The diagnosis of morphea is mainly clinical. Laboratory investigations including histopathology and radiological investigations are helpful in

- Ruling out other differential diagnoses.
- Knowing the disease activity.

S. K. Ghosh (✉) · S. Panja
Department of Dermatology, Venereology, & Leprosy, R.G. Kar Medical College, Kolkata, West Bengal, India

P. Mukherjee
Department of Dermatology, Venereology, & Leprosy, College of Medicine & JNM Hospital, Kalyani, West Bengal, India

P. Agarwal et al. (eds.), *Dermatologist's Handbook of Autoimmune Connective Tissue Diseases*, https://doi.org/10.1007/978-981-95-0524-1_17

Table 17.1 Investigations needed in morphea

Investigation	Interpretation
Dermoscopy	Whitish fibrotic beams, structureless or network-like pigment structures and linear branching vessels
Complete blood count	Rise in eosinophil count, ESR and CRP, to rule out systemic autoimmune disease
Skin biopsy for histopathology	Histopathologically morphea is indistinguishable with systemic sclerosis. Few differentiating features between the two include: Inflammatory cells are more prominent in morphea Changes of sclerosis are seen in the papillary dermis in morphea and in the reticular dermis and subcutis in systemic sclerosis
Serum ANA	ANA, although not currently recommended, but may be positive in 18–68% patients. ENAs found positive are as follows: *Anti ssDNA:* suggests active disease and deeper involvement *Anti-histone:* associated with functional limitations in linear morphea, disease burden, joint contracture, linear subtype *SSA and SSB:* cutaneous changes—hypopigmentation and tightness and neurological changes like paresthesia and carpal tunnel syndrome *Anticentromere*: painful lesions, subcutaneous atrophy, joint contracture *Anti-Sm (smith)*: Shiny skin and pigmentary changes (hypo/hyper) *RA factor*: Associated with joint involvement (arthritis)
Radiological investigations	These are needed in patients with lesions extending beyond dermis. *Ultrasonography (USG):* Helps in evaluating tissue thickness, loss of subcutaneous fat and muscle. *Sun sign* is a classic ultrasound sign for morphea, consists of a hyperechogenic halo surrounding superficial subcutaneous veins of the extremities in transverse view *MRI:* Recommended in patients with morphea affecting the head and neck (rule out asymptomatic intracranial abnormalities) *Reflectance confocal microscopy (RCM), optical coherence tomography (OCT), high-definition optical coherence tomography (HD-OCT):* These are real-time non-invasive imaging techniques
Thermography	It helps in the identification of active morphea variants. Its sensitivity and specificity are 80.7% and 86.3%, respectively

- Assessing depth of involvement.
- Planning effective therapeutic strategies.

The investigations which should be done in patients with morphea are summarized in Table 17.1. The details and interpretation of the various investigations are mentioned in Chap. 4.

17.2 Goals of Treatment

- To arrest lesion expansion and prevent development of new lesions.
- To minimize functional impairment and maximize cosmetic improvement.

General Management

- Counseling regarding the importance of adherence to the treatment regime as some subsets of the disease are chronic and relapsing.

- Use of moisturizers to soften and improve the feel of the skin.
- Avoid long, hot baths as it may lead to further drying of the skin.

Specific Management [4–7]
The therapeutic modality used depends on the disease activity, depth of involvement, and disease progression.

17.3 Medical Therapies

17.3.1 Topical Therapy

For superficial, localized disease.

17.3.1.1 Corticosteroids
High potency corticosteroids are first line of treatment for solitary or limited number of plaques. They can be used under occlusion also, but precaution should be taken against steroid-induced atrophy.

17.3.1.2 Intralesional Corticosteroids
Triamcinolone acetonide in a concentration of 10 mg/mL may be given at the active edges to halt progression.

17.3.1.3 Calcineurin Inhibitors
Tacrolimus 0.1% ointment has shown efficacy in early inflamed lesions. Established sclerotic lesions do not respond well to calcineurin inhibitors.

17.3.1.4 Vitamin D Derivatives
Calcipotriol/calcipotriene ointment either alone or in combination with corticosteroids is effective in inflammatory stage.

17.3.1.5 Imiquimod
In pediatric cases, imiquimod 5% cream has been found to be effective but precludes its use due to possible ulceration of the lesions.

17.4 Systemic Therapy

17.4.1 Immunosuppressive Therapy

It is preferred for multiple, superficial, generalized, rapidly progressive, and deep morphea.

17.4.1.1 Methotrexate
It is used in a dose of 0.6 mg/kg/week for children and 15–25 mg/week in adults as oral dose or subcutaneous injections for 12–24 months. It can be used alone, but in

early stages of development, its use in combination with systemic glucocorticosteroids is seen to be more beneficial.

17.4.1.2 Corticosteroids

Systemic corticosteroids may be used in rapidly progressive disease, both generalized and deep localized morphea. It can be used in daily oral dose (0.5–2 mg/kg/day) or as intravenous pulse of methylprednisolone (30 mg/kg day, max 1 g) on 3 consecutive days/month for at least 3–6 months. Oral dose can be given for 2–4 weeks followed by tapering.

17.4.1.3 Mycophenolate Mofetil

It has been found to be effective for disease refractory to methotrexate or in patients intolerant or having contraindications to methotrexate. Maximum dose used is 1.5 g twice daily.

17.4.1.4 Cyclosporine

It has been seen to reduce activity in early stages at a dose ranging from 1.2 to 3 mg/kg/day.

17.4.1.5 Hydroxychloroquine

Though it was seen to have some efficacy in the treatment of morphea, the latest recommendations do not mention hydroxychloroquine any long.

17.4.2 Phototherapy

It is advisable for localized disease as well as non-progressive generalized disease. UVA and UVA1 have longer wavelength which leads to deeper penetration and are preferred mode of phototherapy in morphea, but their limited availability restricts their use. Their use is also limited in cases with fascial, muscular, or joint involvement. Addition of oral psoralens enhances the efficacy. Narrow band UVB, targeted phototherapy, and extracorporeal photochemotherapy have also been used.

17.5 Newer Small Molecules and Biological Drugs

Various drugs have been found to be effective in refractory and pansclerotic morphea (Table 17.2). However, only limited evidence is present for their use.

Table 17.2 Newer drugs and their mechanism of action

Drug	Mechanism of action
Tofacitinib, ruxolitinib	JAK STAT pathway inhibition
Tocilizumab	Anti IL-6 monoclonal antibody
Everolimus	mTOR inhibitor
Infliximab	Anti TNFα monoclonal antibody

17.6 Surgical

Done mainly in linear morphea. Epiphysiodesis of the unaffected limb to adjust limb length inequality is an option. Plastic surgery can be done to correct the cosmetic deformity in both en coup de sabre and progressive facial hemi atrophy.

Outline of specific management of active and inactive morphea is depicted in Figs. 17.1 and 17.2, respectively [8].

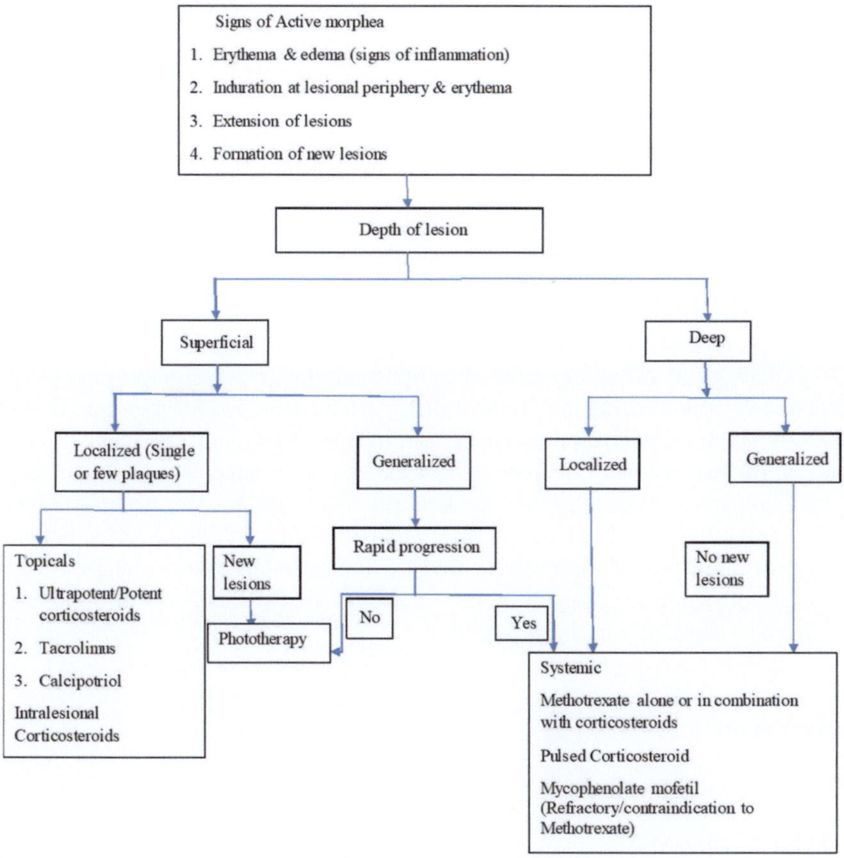

Fig. 17.1 Specific treatment of active morphea

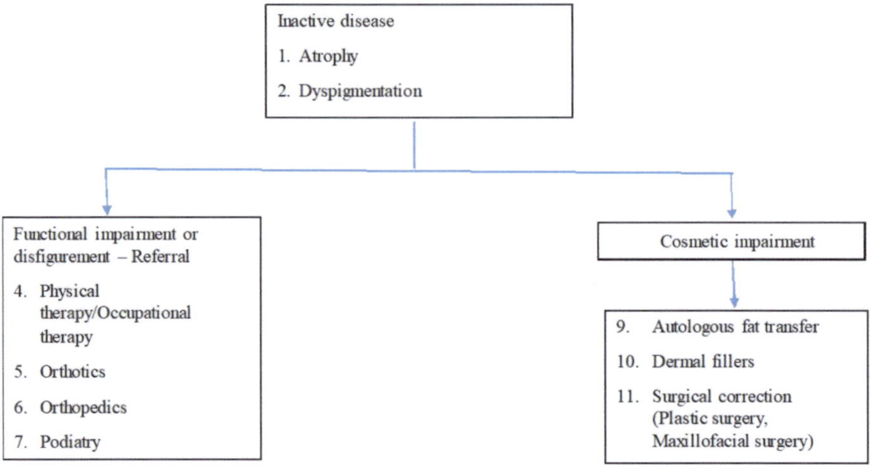

Fig. 17.2 Management of inactive morphea

17.7 Conclusion

The primary goals of management of morphea are to arrest lesion progression and prevent new lesion formation. Topical therapies are effective for localized disease, while systemic immunosuppressive agents, including methotrexate and corticosteroids, form the mainstay of treatment in extensive or rapidly progressive forms. Phototherapy is a valuable adjunct, particularly in non-progressive generalized morphea. Emerging biological agents and small molecule inhibitors offer hope for refractory cases, though their use is currently limited by insufficient long-term data. Surgical correction remains an option in select cases with structural or cosmetic deformities, especially in linear morphea.

References

1. Khatri S, Torok KS, Mirizio E, Liu C, Astakhova K. Autoantibodies in morphea: an update. Front Immunol. 2019;10:1487. https://doi.org/10.3389/fimmu.2019.01487. PMID: 31354701; PMCID: PMC6634257.
2. Torres JE, Sánchez JL. Histopathologic differentiation between localized and systemic scleroderma. Am J Dermatopathol. 1998;20(3):242–5. https://doi.org/10.1097/00000372-199806000-00003.
3. Papara C, De Luca DA, Bieber K, Vorobyev A, Ludwig RJ. Morphea: the 2023 update. Front Med. 2023;10:1108623.
4. George R, George A, Kumar TS. Update on management of morphea (localized scleroderma) in children. Indian Dermatol Online J. 2020;11(2):135–45.
5. Narbutt J, Hołdrowicz A, Lesiak A. Morphea—selected local treatment methods and their effectiveness. Reumatologia. 2017;55:305–13.

6. Pope E, Doria AS, Theriault M, Mohanta A, Laxer RM. Topical imiquimod 5% cream for pediatric plaque morphea: a prospective, multiple-baseline, open-label pilot study. Dermatology. 2011;223:363–9.
7. Zulian F, Culpo R, Sperotto F, Anton J, Avcin T, Baildam EM, et al. Consensus-based recommendations for the management of juvenile localised scleroderma. Ann Rheum Dis. 2019;78:1019–24.
8. Zwischenberger BA, Jacobe HT. A systematic review of morphea treatments and therapeutic algorithm. J Am Acad Dermatol. 2011;65(5):925–41.

Management of Dermatomyositis

18

Bela J. Shah

Abstract

The management of dermatomyositis is complex and needs to be tailored according to age, severity of muscle and skin, as well as systemic involvement. Systemic corticosteroids form the mainstay of therapy for myositis, supported by steroid-sparing immunosuppressive agents such as methotrexate, mycophenolate mofetil, or azathioprine. Cutaneous lesions often respond very well to antimalarials and topical agents, though recalcitrant cases may sometimes require systemic immunosuppressives or biologic therapies. Emerging treatments include Janus kinase inhibitors like tofacitinib and other biologics, and they show promise in refractory cases.

Keywords

Dermatomyositis · Corticosteroids · Biologics

Dermatomyositis and polymyositis are long-term inflammatory muscle diseases, causing muscle weakness and disability. This chapter will outline the necessary investigations required to be carried out in a patient with dermatomyositis and overview of pharmacotherapy.

B. J. Shah (✉)
Department of Skin & VD, GCS Medical College, Hospital and Research Centre, Ahmedabad, Gujarat, India

P. Agarwal et al. (eds.), *Dermatologist's Handbook of Autoimmune Connective Tissue Diseases*, https://doi.org/10.1007/978-981-95-0524-1_18

18.1 Investigations

The patients suspected to have dermatomyositis need to undergo following investigations (details mentioned in the Chaps. 3 and 4) (Box 18.1).

Box 18.1: Summary of Investigations
- CBC.
- ESR, CRP.
- Urine-routine, 24 h urinary protein.
- Liver and renal function tests.
- Serum CPK, LDH.
- ANA profile.
- Skin biopsy.
- Barium swallow, upper GI endoscopy (as required).
- Pulmonary function tests (as required).
- High-resolution CT lung (as required).

18.2 Various Auto-antibodies Found in DM and Their Implications

The panel of myositis-associated antibodies needs to be ordered separately than ANA immunoblot assay. Table 18.1 gives information about the dermatomyositis autoantibodies [1]:

1. *Myositis-associated autoantibodies (MAA):* anti-PM Scl, anti-U1, anti-U2, anti U3-RNP, anti-Hu anti-SSA/anti-Ro, and anti-Sjogren's syndrome B (anti-SSB)/anti-La autoantibodies.

Table 18.1 Various myositis specific antibodies and their implications

Antibodies	Clinical characteristics	Treatment response and prognosis
Anti-Mi-5	Subacute onset of classic dermatomyositis, typical skin involvement	Good response to corticosteroids
Anti-MDAS	Severe skin involvement, can present as amyopathic form, rapidly progressive ILD, vasculopathy	Poorest survival
Anti-NXP-2	Mild to moderate weakness, classic skin rash, calcinosis	Good response to treatment, monitor for malignancy
Anti-SAE	Mild to moderate muscle involvement, typical skin findings	Monitor for malignancy
Anti-TIF1	Hyperkeratotic papules, telangiectasias, hypopigmentation	Monitor for malignancy

2. *Myositis-specific autoantibodies (MSA):* anti-Mi-2, anti-melanoma differentiation-associated protein-5 (anti-MDA-5), anti-nuclear matrix protein-2 (anti-NXP-2), anti-TIF-1, and anti-small ubiquitin-like modifier activating enzyme (anti-SAE)-1/2.

18.3 Principles of Treatment of DM

- Treatment of dermatomyositis depends on the age of the patient, degree of myositis, cutaneous lesions, any systemic involvement, and association with malignancy. Therapy aims at increasing muscle strength to improve daily activity, improving cutaneous and treating systemic complications if any.
- Collaborative management under rheumatologist, dermatologist, neurologist, and pulmonologist is critical for patients with multisystem involvement.
- Cutaneous DM has discordant treatment response with muscle disease, with recalcitrant skin disease continuing years after muscle disease is in remission.

18.3.1 General Management

- Screening for malignancy: As treatment of the cancer may reduce disease severity or even induce disease remission.
- Photoprotection: First step in management though 60% of cases are minimally photosensitive.
- Avoidance of direct sunlight exposure, wearing full-sleeve clothes dress, using umbrella or broad-brim hats. Proper use of broad-spectrum sunscreen 15 min before going out in the sun and reapplication as directed by physician.

18.3.2 Topical Therapy for Skin Lesions in DM

- Topical agents are preferred for cutaneous limited lesions of DM.
- Topical corticosteroids: Class I or II creams and ointments can be used with or without occlusion. They reduce pruritus, erythema, and scaling and can also be tried to mitigate the problem of nail fold sensitivity [2].
- Topical calcineurin inhibitors such as tacrolimus 0.1% ointment or pimecrolimus 1% cream can also be used; safe to use over face without concern for atrophy or hypopigmentation [3, 4].

18.3.3 Systemic Therapy for DM

18.3.3.1 Antimalarials

Hydroxychloroquine (3.5–6.5 mg/kg per day) or chloroquine (250 mg daily) is the first line of treatment for cutaneous lesions [1]. Antimalarials also ameliorate mild symptoms of inflammatory arthritis but are ineffective against myositis and interstitial lung disease.

18.3.3.2 Corticosteroids

Corticosteroids are the first-line agent for DM-associated myopathy. They reduce the disease activity and improve muscle strength. They also reduce long-term disability and mortality [5].

- They can be given as daily oral dose (0.5–1 mg/kg) or in severe disease as intravenous pulse therapy (1000 mg of methylprednisolone for 3 consecutive days).
- Oral steroids should be tapered slowly once the disease activity is controlled and may be given for a period of 6–12 months.
- They should never be used as a monotherapy and have no significant benefit in postmyopathic cutaneous lesions.

18.3.3.3 Oral Immunosuppressive Agents

They should be started along with systemic steroids as steroid sparing agents [5].

- Methotrexate (20–25 mg/week)—It should be avoided in patients having interstitial lung disease.
- Mycophenolate mofetil (MMF, 1.5 g bid).
- Azathioprine (2.5 mg/kg/day).
- Cyclophosphamide-IV cyclophosphamide (0.5–1.0 g/m^2 IV monthly) can be combined with pulse dose of steroids for severe life-threatening disease.

All these drugs have beneficial effects over the cutaneous lesions also in addition to myositis.

18.3.3.4 Rituximab

Rituximab is advocated as a third-line therapy for DM [2].

- It is useful in myositis, especially with anti-Jo 1 and anti-Mi-2 autoantibodies.
- It is useful in recalcitrant cutaneous lesions and can be used as first-line therapy for vasculitic skin lesions associated with anti-MDA5 and anti-NXP-2 antibodies, as well as myositis not responding to standard therapy of systemic corticosteroids and immunosuppressive agents.

18.3.3.5 Intravenous Immunoglobulin

It is the single most effective agent with relatively quick action and is preferred in acutely ill or severely declining patients with dysphagia or respiratory involvement.

Dose of IVIg is 2 g/kg body weight divided over 3–5 days [2].

They also work well in refractory skin lesions, calcinosis cutis, and myositis not responding to even rituximab.

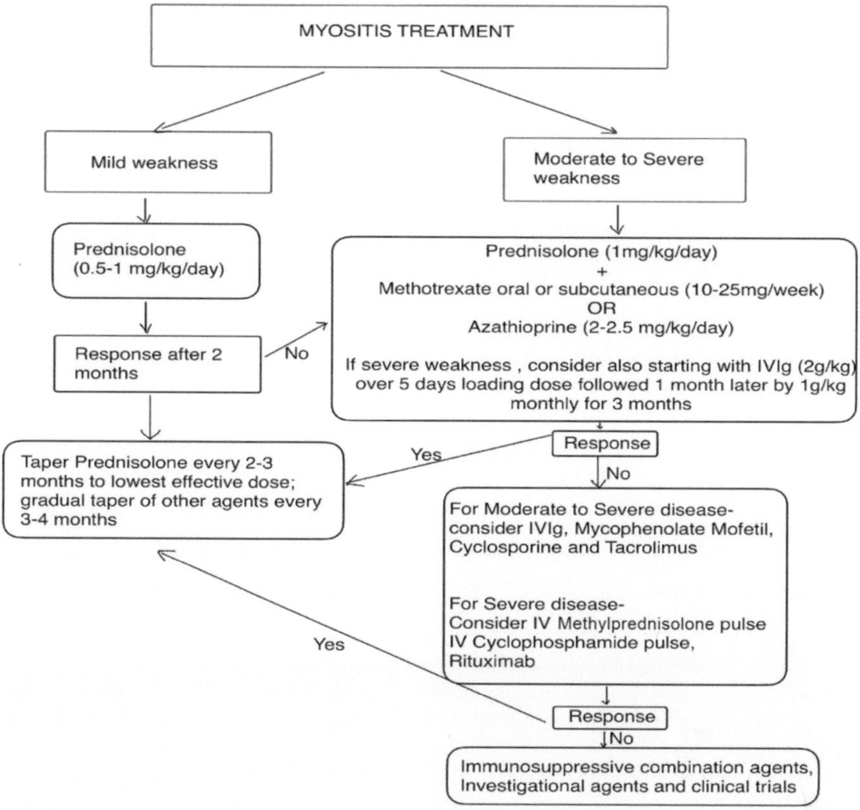

Fig. 18.1 Treatment approach toward dermatomyositis

Early intervention helps in reducing the incidence of calcinosis cutis. Though the lesions are often resistant to therapy, drugs which have been tried with variable results include bisphosphonates, diltiazem, minocycline, and colchicine. Surgical excision may be advised in cases with few lesions [6].

18.3.3.6 Janus Kinase Inhibitors

Both tofacitinib and baricitinib have shown promising results in refractory cutaneous lesions [7].

18.3.3.7 Other Biologics

Many biologic agents are being explored for the treatment of recalcitrant cases of dermatomyositis and include anakinra, abatacept, alemtuzumab, anifrolumab, belimumab, eculizumab, and tocilizumab [2, 8, 9].

A stepwise approach to treatment of DM is summarized in Fig. 18.1.

18.4 Conclusion

While systemic corticosteroids remain the cornerstone for treating myopathy, combination therapy with immunosuppressants enhances treatment efficacy and at the same time minimizes steroid-related adverse effects. Cutaneous lesions are often more resistant and persistent and demand significant therapeutic attention with antimalarials, topical agents (including corticosteroids and calcineurin inhibitors), and advanced immunomodulators. For refractory or rapidly progressive disease, intravenous immunoglobulin, biologics, and emerging agents like Janus kinase inhibitors have been shown to offer promising results.

References

1. Marasandra Ramesh H, Gude SS, Venugopal S, Peddi NC, Gude SS, Vuppalapati S. The role of myositis-specific autoantibodies in the dermatomyositis spectrum. Cureus. 2022;14(3):e22978. https://doi.org/10.7759/cureus.22978. PMID: 35415038; PMCID: PMC8990210.
2. Waldman R, DeWane ME, Lu J. Dermatomyositis: diagnosis and treatment. J Am Acad Dermatol. 2020;82(2):283–96.
3. Hollar CB, Jorizzo JL. Topical tacrolimus 0.1% ointment for refractory skin disease in dermatomyositis: a pilot study. J Dermatol Treat. 2004;15(1):35–9.
4. Kim JE, Jeong MG, Lee HE, Ko JY, Ro YS. Successful treatment of cutaneous lesions of dermatomyositis with topical pimecrolimus. Ann Dermatol. 2011;23(3):348–51.
5. Joffe MM, Love LA, Leff RL, et al. Drug therapy of the idiopathic inflammatory myopathies: predictors of response to prednisone, azathioprine, and methotrexate and a comparison of their efficacy. Am J Med. 1993;94(4):379–87.
6. Traineau H, Aggarwal R, Monfort JB, et al. Treatment of calcinosis cutis in systemic sclerosis and dermatomyositis: a review of the literature. J Am Acad Dermatol. 2020;82(2):317–25.
7. Kurtzman DJ, Wright NA, Lin J, et al. Tofacitinib citrate for refractory cutaneous dermatomyositis: an alternative treatment. JAMA Dermatol. 2016;152(8):944–5.
8. Shaw KS, Hashemi KB, Castillo RL, Rainone E, Ho AW, Kahn PJ, Oza VS, Femia A, Vleugels RA. Anifrolumab in recalcitrant cutaneous dermatomyositis: a multicenter retrospective cohort study. J Am Acad Dermatol. 2024;12:S0190-9622(24)02609-4.
9. Liu Y, Li Y, Shen T, Zhang H, Luo S, Zhang Q, Dang X, Li X, Long H. Belimumab ameliorates symptoms and disease activity in patients with dermatomyositis and juvenile dermatomyositis refractory to standard therapy: a retrospective observational study. J Am Acad Dermatol. 2024;91(3):524–7.

Management of Sjögren's Syndrome

19

Sapan C. Pandya and Kunal Chandwar

Abstract

Sjögren's syndrome is a chronic autoimmune condition which usually presents to rheumatologists and less commonly to dermatologists. Still, a dermatologist should be aware of the investigations and treatment strategies for the disease. Apart from investigating for antinuclear antibodies, the patients need a detailed ophthalmic and salivary gland evaluation for reduced secretions. A multidisciplinary approach is warranted and includes lifestyle modifications, symptomatic relief of sicca symptoms, and systemic therapy tailored to organ involvement. This chapter discusses the management of Sjögren's syndrome including the investigations and pharmacotherapy by an experienced rheumatologist.

Keywords

Sjögren's syndrome · Investigations · Dry eyes · Dry mouth

19.1 Investigations

Apart from the specific tests outlined in Table 19.1, few patients of Sjögren's syndrome may have raised ESRs, leucopenia, low platelet count, high globulins in blood, and rheumatoid factor positivity. This is the subset with higher inflammatory burden, and more extraglandular complications of Sjögren's syndrome and hence more likely to evolve into a lymphoma [1].

S. C. Pandya (✉)
Department of Rheumatology, SVPIMSR, Smt NHL Municipal Medical College, Ahmedabad, India

K. Chandwar
Department of Clinical Immunology and Rheumatology, Sanjay Gandhi Postgraduate Institute of Medical Sciences, Lucknow, India

P. Agarwal et al. (eds.), *Dermatologist's Handbook of Autoimmune Connective Tissue Diseases*, https://doi.org/10.1007/978-981-95-0524-1_19

Table 19.1 Investigations needed in Sjögren's syndrome [2–4]

Test	How it is done	Sensitivity and specificity
Schirmer's	Filter paper strip inserted into lower eyelid and then wetness measured over 5 min: <5 mm for dry eye	76.9% and 4–72%, respectively
Lissamine green for ocular surface	5–10 microliter (μL) or up to 20 of the dye instilled into fornix of the eye using strip and patient is asked to blink. It stains the areas that are dry—Rose Bengal can also be used	64.3% and 81.7%, respectively
Salivary flow rate	All saliva dribbling into a container is collected for 15 min and then measured: normal is more than 1.5 mL. The stimulated version uses gum or citric acid as salivary stimulants	56.1% and 80.7%, respectively
Salivary gland ultrasound (US)	Non-invasive method—almost replacing others—glandular inhomogeneity and hypoechoic areas suggest inflammation; there are validated scoring systems now	95% and 98%, respectively
MRI salivary glands	Multiple hypo- and hyper-intense areas (salt and pepper) suggest inflammation, and in more advanced stages, cystic changes are seen	Same as US; hence most groups use US
Salivary gland biopsy	From lower lip 5–7 accessory glands are sampled—focus scores are counted; one FS is aggregate of >50 lymphocytes per 4 mm^2. Scoring systems are validated for the same	82.4% and 86.2%, respectively
Anti-Ro	By immunoblot; can also be done by ELISA	69–77% and 83–95% (with focus score 1 or more)
Anti-La	By immunoblot; can also be done by ELISA	39–44% sensitivity
ANA	By immunofluorescence	50% sensitivity

19.2 Treatment

To a dermatologist, patients with Sjögren's syndrome might present with dry skin, palpable purpura (rarely cryoglobulinemic), or anti-Ro-associated subacute cutaneous lupus erythematosus like skin rash. Multidisciplinary approach is essential as Sjögren's syndrome usually has extra-cutaneous involvement also in terms of joint pains, parotitis, renal tubular acidosis, etc.

19.2.1 General Measures

The therapy includes lifestyle modifications in addition to organ targeted therapy.

Lifestyle modifications include avoidance of the following:

- Smoking.
- Aerated beverages.

Table 19.2 Treatment for sicca symptoms in the eyes and mouth [5, 6]

Drug	Adverse effects
Dry eyes	
Artificial tears (carboxy and hydroxy methylcellulose, hyaluronic acid)	Preservative can cause conjunctivitis, subconjuctival fibrosis, ocular surface changes
Topical steroids	Cataract/infection/raised intraocular tension. Mild systemic absorption will be there
Topical cyclosporine	Stinging sensation
Autologous serum therapy	Infection
Topical N-acetylcysteine	Stinging sensation, sulfur odor
Topical Lifitegrast (LFA-1 antagonist)	Irritation, reduced visual acuity
Dry mouth	
Saliva substitute	Sticky, unpleasant sensation
Topical antifungal	Burning sensation
Systemic therapy	
Pilocarpine and cevimeline *For dry mouth > dry eyes*	Sweating, urinary frequency, flushing, excessive salivation, giddiness, abdominal pain, etc.

- Dry environments like air conditioning/high winds.
- Continuous work on laptops/computers.
- Excessive screen time.
- Anticholinergic drugs.
- Improper dental hygiene.

19.2.2 Treatment of Sicca Symptoms in the Eye and Mouth

Due to impairment of the quality of life, treatment for dry eyes and mouth forms a cornerstone in the management of patients with Sjögren's syndrome and is summarized in Table 19.2.

19.2.3 Systemic Therapy for Organ Involvement [7–9]

After assessment of the disease activity, systemic therapy depends on the extent of organ involvement (Figs. 19.1 and 19.2).

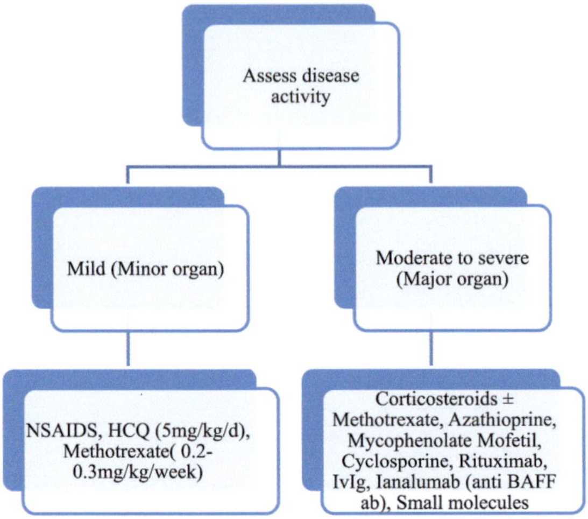

Fig. 19.1 Systemic management of Sjögren's syndrome

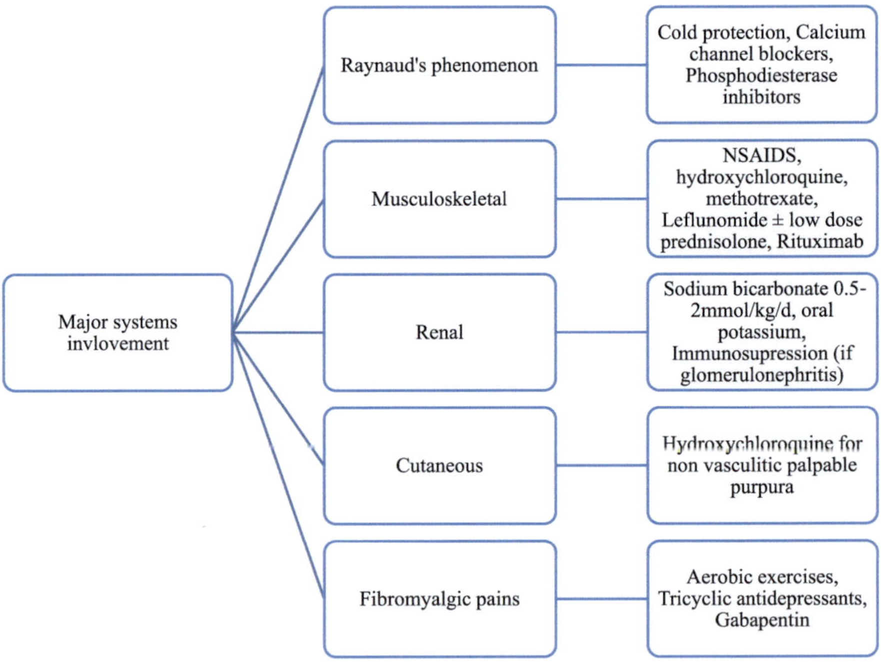

Fig. 19.2 Systemic therapy according to major organ involvement

References

1. Quartuccio L, Isola M, Baldini C, Priori R, Bartoloni Bocci E, Carubbi F, et al. Biomarkers of lymphoma in Sjogren's syndrome and evaluation of the lymphoma risk in prelymphomatous conditions: results of a multicenter study. J Autoimmun. 2014;51:75e80.
2. Mavragani CP, Moutsopoulos H. Sjogren's syndrome. CMAJ. 2014;186(15):E579–86.
3. Lorenzon M, Spina E, Tulipano Di Franco F, Giovannini I, De Vita S, Zabotti A. Salivary gland ultrasound in primary Sjögren's syndrome: current and future perspectives. Open Access Rheumatol. 2022;14:147–60. https://doi.org/10.2147/OARRR.S284763. PMID: 36072437; PMCID: PMC9444027.
4. Lorenzon M, Spina E, Di Franco FT, Giovannini I, De Vita S, Zabotti A. Salivary gland ultrasound in primary Sjögren's syndrome: current and future perspectives. Open Access Rheumatol. 2022;14:147–60.
5. Sall K, Stevenson OD, Mundorf TK, Reis BL. Two multicenter, randomized studies of the efficacy and safety of cyclosporine ophthalmic emulsion in moderate to severe dry eye disease. CsA Phase 3 Study Group. Ophthalmology. 2000;107:631.
6. Papas AS, Sherrer YS, Charney M, et al. Successful treatment of dry mouth and dry eye symptoms in Sjögren's syndrome patients with oral pilocarpine: a randomized, placebo-controlled, dose-adjustment study. J Clin Rheumatol. 2004;10:169.
7. Seror R, Bowman SJ, Brito-Zeron P, et al. EULAR Sjögren's syndrome disease activity index (ESSDAI): a user guide. RMD Open. 2015;1:e000022. https://doi.org/10.1136/rmdopen-2014-000022.
8. Gottenberg JE, Ravaud P, Puéchal X, Le Guern V, Sibilia J, Goeb V, Larroche C, et al. Effects of hydroxychloroquine on symptomatic improvement in primary Sjögren syndrome: the JOQUER randomized clinical trial. JAMA. 2014;312(3):249–58.
9. Sada PR, Isenberg D, Ciurtin C. Biologic treatment in Sjogren's syndrome. Rheumatology. 2015;54:219–30.

Management of Mixed Connective Tissue Disease, Overlap Syndrome, and Undifferentiated Connective Tissue Disease

20

Puja Srivastava

Abstract

Connective tissue diseases (CTDs) are multisystem autoimmune disorders with a chronic relapsing and remitting course. Due to the absence of definitive diagnostic tests, their diagnosis essentially relies on evolving classification criteria. Undifferentiated CTD (UCTD) and overlap syndromes frequently present with overlapping features of well defined CTDs, while mixed connective tissue disease (MCTD) is a distinct entity. Although a number of UCTD cases may never progress into a defined CTD, early progression, usually within 5 years, is common. Management is based on symptoms, severity of organ involvement, and treatment protocols of the primary CTDs. Pulmonary hypertension is one of the leading causes of mortality in MCTD, while complications such as Raynaud's phenomenon, ILD, and hematologic and renal involvement also contribute to morbidity and mortality.

In CTDs, regular monitoring for disease progression and disease as well as treatment-related complications is essential. Prognosis of overlap CTDs is usually better than primary forms, especially in patients with high U1-RNP antibodies. The goals of therapy should be symptom control, prevention and control organ damage, and reduction of treatment-related side effects.

20.1 Introduction

Connective tissue diseases (CTDs) are multisystem disorders with a plethora of different signs and symptoms. Up to 10% to 20% of patients diagnosed with undifferentiated connective tissue disease (UCTD) will never progress into a

P. Srivastava (✉)
Division of Rheumatology, Allergy and Immunology, Star Clinics, Ahmedabad, India

P. Agarwal et al. (eds.), *Dermatologist's Handbook of Autoimmune Connective Tissue Diseases*, https://doi.org/10.1007/978-981-95-0524-1_20

well-defined CTD. The rate of progression into a defined CTD is the highest within the first 5 years of disease onset and then decreases significantly over time. Management of CTDs requires an early and timely diagnosis and is guided by the type of organ involvement.

The diagnosis of these disorders is based on classification criteria, which include both clinical and immunological aspects of the disease. At present, there are six well-defined CTDs, based on their specific clinical and immunological features. They are systemic lupus erythematosus (SLE), Sjögren's syndrome, systemic sclerosis, dermatomyositis, polymyositis, and rheumatoid arthritis [1]. All six of these classic CTDs are descriptive syndromes based on consensus classification criteria but lack a gold standard diagnostic test or criteria. These criteria are modified from time to time as new knowledge accumulates.

20.2 Investigations

The investigations which should be carried out in patients with suspected MCTD, UCTD or overlap syndromes are outlined in Table 20.1 [2–6]. Certain antibodies are seen more commonly in specific overlap syndromes and are mentioned in Table 20.2 [7, 8].

Table 20.1 Investigations in suspected MCTD, UCTD and overlap syndromes

Routine screening tests	Complete blood count CRP ESR Serum creatinine Thyroid-stimulating hormone Urinalysis with microscopic analysis SGOT/SGPT
ANA/ENA	Anti-Ro/SS-A and Anti SS-B Anti-U1-RNP Anti jo1 Anti-smith Anti-mi2 Anti-Ku Anti-scl70 (topoisomerase antibody) Anti-chromatin Anti-histone
As and when required for assessment of disease	Complement components (C3, C4, CH50) Creatine kinase Aldolase Anti-cyclic citrullinated peptide (CCP)/RA Factor Pulmonary function tests Electrocardiography Schirmer test in patients with dry eye; APLA Antibody Profile

(continued)

Table 20.1 (continued)

Imaging	*Chest radiography* Pleural or pericardial effusion Longstanding pulmonary hypertension Cardiomegaly Interstitial lung disease *Chest computed tomography* Interstitial lung disease *Ultrasonography salivary glands* To differentiate between undifferentiated connective tissue disease and Sjögren's syndrome

Table 20.2 Specific overlap syndrome and associated with auto-antibodies

Autoantibody	Overlap syndrome
Anti-U1-snRNP Ab	MCTD (clinical features of SLE, myositis, scleroderma, and RA)
Anti-PM-Scl Ab	Myositis (polymyositis) and systemic sclerosis (Raynaud's)
Anti-synthetase Ab	Features of myositis, arthritis, interstitial lung disease
Anti-SSA/B with RF and anti-CCP Ab	Features of RA and Sjögren's

20.3 Treatment of Connective Tissue Diseases [9]

Management of UCTDs and overlap syndromes has not been studied in randomized controlled trials (RCTs). Hence, there are no validated outcome measures for assessing activity or damage in overlap CTDs and MCTD. At present, majority of studies use tools designated for assessment of primary CTDs like SLE, SSc, PM/DM, etc. Similarly, recommendations for management are based on the conventional treatment protocols used for primary CTDs like RA, SLE, systemic sclerosis, etc. For example, inflammatory arthritis is managed on the lines of rheumatoid arthritis, while Raynaud's phenomenon is managed on the lines of systemic sclerosis. The clinical features of CTDs can change over time; hence the management strategies may need frequent readjustments in medications and close follow-ups.

The goals of therapy for UCTD overlap syndromes and MCTD are to control disease related symptoms, to preserve organ functions, and to reduce the disease or treatment-related complications and damage accrual in different organs.

Medical therapy targets control of disease activity in general, and management plan is based on the type and severity of the specific organ involvement (Table 20.3). Complicated Raynaud's phenomenon and digital ischemia are the main causes of morbidity, while pulmonary arterial hypertension is the main cause of mortality in UCTD/MCTD spectrum of illnesses. Moderate and severe organ involvements (such as hematological, renal, severe interstitial lung disease (ILD) or neurological

Table 20.3 Management of overlap syndromes

System involved	Clinical problems	Suggested treatments
Constitutional features	Fatigue, arthralgia fever	NSAIDs Anti-malarial Low-dose prednisone (<10 mg/day)
Vascular problems	Raynaud's phenomenon	Cold protection Calcium channel blockers PD4 inhibitors (tadalafil/sildenafil)
	Digital gangrene	Vasodilators PD4i, ER antagonists Prostacyclin infusions Short-term anticoagulation Digital sympathectomy (painful refractory cases)
Musculo-skeletal problems	Arthritis	NSAIDs Anti-malarial Methotrexate and other conventional DMARDs Rituximab in refractory cases
	Myositis	Prednisone (0.5–1 mg/kg) in tapering doses Methotrexate Azathioprine Mycophenolate mofetil In refractory cases Rituximab IVIG
	Osteoporosis	Calcium/vitamin D supplements Teriparatide Denosumab Bisphosphonates Avoid long-term glucocorticoids
Cardiopulmonary problems	Pericarditis/pleuritis	NSAIDs Prednisone (short course)
	Pulmonary hypertension	Vasodilators: PD4i, ER antagonists Immuno-modulator: Prednisone and cyclophosphamide/mycophenolate mofetil
	Myocarditis	Prednisone Cyclophosphamide
	Interstitial lung disease (ILD)	Prednisone Cyclophosphamide Mycophenolate mofetil Rituximab (with progressive ILD)

(continued)

Table 20.3 (continued)

System involved	Clinical problems	Suggested treatments
Hematological problems	Autoimmune hemolytic anemia (AIHA) thrombocytopenia	High-dose prednisone Azathioprine Cyclosporine Mycophenolate mofetil IVIG (refractory cases) Thrombopoietic growth factors (eltrombopag) can be added in thrombocytopenia
	Thrombotic thrombo-cytopenic purpura (TTP)	High-dose prednisone Rituximab Plasma exchange Fresh frozen plasma Platelet concentrate infusions
Gastro-intestinal problems	Dyspepsia/gastro-esophageal reflux	H2 antagonists Proton pump inhibitors Prokinetic agents (look for *H. pylori* infection in recalcitrant cases)
	Intestinal dysmotility	Prokinetic agents like itopride, metoclopramide
Neurological problems	Trigeminal neuralgia	No definitive treatment options Anti-epileptics (ox-carbamazepine) Others: Gabapentin/tricyclic anti-depressants
	Sensori-neural hearing loss (SNHL)	Short course of high-dose oral prednisone (1 mg/kg and taper)
	Aseptic meningitis	Stop NSIADs, short burst of oral prednisone (40–60 mg/day)
Renal problems	Membranous glomerulonephritis	Mild: ACE inhibitor, BP control Moderate/severe: Prednisone, pulse cyclophosphamide, mycophenolate mofetil, rituximab (steroids alone are rarely helpful)
	Scleroderma-like renal crisis	ACE inhibitors, Direct renin inhibitors and supportive care

PD4i phosphodiesterase inhibitors like sildenafil, tadalafil, etc.
ER antagonists endothelin receptor antagonists like bosentan and ambrisentan

manifestations) are not very uncommon, and may sometimes progress to life-threatening conditions. If all patients with idiopathic nonspecific interstitial pneumonia are screened, around 88% of the patients with may meet the diagnostic criteria for UCTD/CTD Spectrum of diseases.

Patients should be evaluated at regular intervals for these complications; early detection and intervention are the key to effective management. Treating physicians should be vigilant for treatment-related complications like recurrent atypical infections, steroid-induced myopathy, accelerated osteoporosis, and avascular necrosis of bones in patients treated with long-term immunomodulatory therapies.

20.4 Prognosis and Long-Term Outcome [10–12]

The prognosis of autoimmune overlap CTDs is often better than the established CTDs. For example, patients with overlap SSc and overlap myositis have a better prognosis then primary SSc and primary PM/DM, respectively. Most patients with overlap CTD syndromes have a relatively benign disease course, but the pattern of major organ involvement ultimately dictates the morbidity and mortality of the disease.

There is unequivocal evidence that presence of high titers of U1-RNP antibodies is associated with low prevalence of severe renal and neurological disease, which means that patients with MCTD have better prognosis as compared to lupus. The main cause of mortality in MCTD is pulmonary arterial hypertension, with few reports related to infections and cardiovascular events. According to report by Hajas et al., 5, 10, and 15 year survival rates among patients with MCTD were of 98%, 96%, and 88%, respectively.

20.5 Conclusion

The goals of therapy for undifferentiated, overlap syndromes and mixed connective tissue disease (MCTD) are to control disease-related symptoms and to preserve organ functions. Further goals also are to reduce damage accrual in different organs with a timely diagnosis and treatment. There are no diagnostic tests; diagnosis of these disorders is based on classification criteria. The management of overlap syndromes is based on the usual treatment of the manifested clinical symptoms like arthritis, myositis, Raynaud's, or other systemic complaints in diseases like lupus, rheumatoid arthritis, scleroderma, or inflammatory myositis. The prognosis of undifferentiated and mixed connective tissue disease relies on the degree of organ involvement. Pulmonary hypertension is a major cause of mortality in MCTD; thus all patients should be screened by echocardiograms at regular intervals.

References

1. Bennet RM. Overlap syndromes. In: Kelly's and Firestein textbook of rheumatology, vol. 2. Philadelphia: Elsevier; 2017. p. 1489–511.
2. Mosca M, Tani C, Neri C, Baldini C, Bombardieri S. Undifferentiated connective tissue diseases (UCTD). Autoimmun Rev. 2006;6(1):1–4. [PubMed] [Reference list].
3. Zold E, Szodoray P, Gaal J, Kappelmayer J, Csathy L, Gyimesi E, Zeher M, Szegedi G, Bodolay E. Vitamin D deficiency in undifferentiated connective tissue disease. Arthritis Res Ther. 2008;10(5):R123.
4. González C, Garcia-Berrocal B, Herráez O, Navajo JA, González-Buitrago JM. Anti-nucleosome, anti-chromatin, anti-dsDNA and anti-histone antibody reactivity in systemic lupus erythematosus. Clin Chem Lab Med. 2004;42(3):266–72.
5. Luciano N, Baldini C, Tarantini G, Ferro F, Sernissi F, Varanini V, Donati V, Martini D, Mosca M, Caramella D, Bombardieri S. Ultrasonography of major salivary glands: a highly specific tool for distinguishing primary Sjögren's syndrome from undifferentiated connective tissue diseases. Rheumatology (Oxford). 2015;54(12):2198–204.

6. Ceribelli A, Cavazzana I, Franceschini F, Quinzanini M, Rizzini FL, Cattaneo R. Isotype switching and titer variation of anti-Ro/SSA antibodies over time in 100 patients with undifferentiated connective tissue disease (UCTD). Clin Exp Rheumatol. 2008;26(1):117–20.
7. Belizna C, et al. Anti-Ku antibodies: clinical, genetic and diagnostic insights. Autoimmun Rev. 2010;9(10):691–4. https://doi.org/10.1016/j.autrev.2010.05.020.
8. Pepmueller PH. Undifferentiated connective tissue disease, mixed connective tissue disease, and overlap syndromes in rheumatology. Mo Med. 2016;113(2):136–40. PMID: 27311225; PMCID: PMC6139943.
9. Chernau AK, Leone PM, Swigris JJ. Interstitial pneumonia with autoimmune features and undifferentiated connective tissue disease. Semin Respir Crit Care Med. 2019;40(2):271–7. [PubMed: 31137065].
10. Troyanov Y, Targoff IN, Tremblay JL, et al. Novel classification of idiopathic inflammatory myopathies based on overlap syndrome features and autoantibodies: analysis of 100 French Canadian patients. Medicine (Baltimore). 2005;84(4):231–49.
11. Wanzenrled A, Garalman A, Jordan S, et al. The enigma of mixed connective tissue disease—challenges in routine care. Clin Rheumatol. 2022;41:3503–11.
12. Hajas A, Szodoray P, Nakken B, et al. Clinical course, prognosis, and causes of death in mixed connective tissue disease. J Rheumatol. 2013;40(7):1134–42.

MIX
Papier aus verantwortungsvollen Quellen
Paper from responsible sources
FSC® C105338

If you have any concerns about our products,
you can contact us on
ProductSafety@springernature.com

In case Publisher is established outside the EU,
the EU authorized representative is:
Springer Nature Customer Service Center GmbH
Europaplatz 3, 69115 Heidelberg, Germany

Printed by Libri Plureos GmbH
in Hamburg, Germany